DISCOVER THE POWER OF HERBAL REMEDIES

THE BEGINNER'S GUIDE TO NATURAL MEDICINE REMEDIES FOR DIGESTIVE PROBLEMS, STRESS, INSOMNIA, ALLERGIES, PAINS, LOW ENERGY, AND MORE – A HOLISTIC APPROACH TO BETTER HEALTH

LEAF INSIGHT BOOKS

© Copyright 2024 - All rights reserved.

The content contained within this book may not be reproduced, duplicated or transmitted without direct written permission from the author or the publisher.

Under no circumstances will any blame or legal responsibility be held against the publisher, or author, for any damages, reparation, or monetary loss due to the information contained within this book, either directly or indirectly.

Legal Notice:

This book is copyright protected. It is only for personal use. You cannot amend, distribute, sell, use, quote or paraphrase any part, or the content within this book, without the consent of the author or publisher.

Disclaimer Notice:

Please note the information contained within this document is for educational and entertainment purposes only. All effort has been executed to present accurate, up to date, reliable, complete information. No warranties of any kind are declared or implied. Readers acknowledge that the author is not engaged in the rendering of legal, financial, medical or professional advice. The content within this book has been derived from various sources. Please consult a licensed professional before attempting any techniques outlined in this book.

By reading this document, the reader agrees that under no circumstances is the author responsible for any losses, direct or indirect, that are incurred as a result of the use of the information contained within this document, including, but not limited to, errors, omissions, or inaccuracies.

INTRODUCTION

Meet Akosua, a Ghanaian woman whose journey through pregnancy reflects the deep-rooted reliance on herbal remedies in her community. In Ghana, herbal remedies aren't just alternatives —they are the primary solution, woven intricately into the fabric of everyday life.

From the moment she learned of her pregnancy, she knew that herbs would play a vital role in her prenatal care. In her world, conventional medicine often takes a back seat to the wisdom regarding herbs passed down through generations. Unlike the Western world, where hospitals and pharmacies abound, Akosua's community values herbal knowledge above all else.

Her confidence in herbal remedies isn't merely a matter of preference—it reflects her upbringing and cultural heritage. Her family and community have relied on herbs for healing and wellness for generations. The familiarity with traditional herbs runs deep within her veins, shaping her understanding of health and medicine.

As she navigates through her pregnancy, she finds solace in her profound understanding of these herbal medicines. She knows their benefits, their risks, and their limitations. In her community, there's no need for extensive research or second-guessing—the knowledge of herbs is instinctual, passed down from one generation to the next.

We invite you to a similar journey toward natural healing to harness your knowledge and develop critical techniques in using natural remedies. Welcome to *Discover the Power of Herbal Remedies*.

This book is about the extraordinary power of nature's gifts. You will discover the profound effect of traditional herbs on your well-being and embrace simplicity as you unlock the secrets of herbal remedies.

UNLOCKING THE POWER OF HERBS

Exploring herbal remedies may feel unfamiliar or daunting at first. You may have concerns about their effectiveness or safety, especially if you're accustomed to conventional medicine. It's also natural to wonder how herbs fit into your lifestyle and health journey.

We know that you:

- Feel worried about your well-being due to persistent aches and pains, longer recovery times, and the negative impacts of bad habits on your health.
- Are concerned about worsening mental health. You may feel stressed, anxious, and depressed, and your physical conditions worsen these.
- Feel confused about contradicting and sometimes lacking information about herbal remedies available online.

- Are unsure about your skills and knowledge in making herbal remedies, thinking they are complicated to prepare.
- Lack the time to learn and prepare herbal remedies because of your busy life.

We aim to address your doubts and provide clarity, helping you embrace herbal remedies confidently and efficiently.

WHY DISCOVER THE POWER OF HERBAL REMEDIES?

This book gives you hope when you face ongoing health issues. It encourages you to explore different ways to feel better beyond what you're used to. As you deal with persistent symptoms, you realize waiting for them to go away on their own isn't enough. Choosing herbal remedies becomes essential because you want relief from mental and physical discomfort.

Health problems don't just go away by themselves; thus, taking action is key. If you don't do anything, your symptoms might get worse, both physically and mentally. Turning to herbal remedies isn't just an option anymore; you need to do something to feel better and take care of yourself.

BENEFITS OF DISCOVERING THE POWER OF HERBAL REMEDIES

Learning about herbal remedies for the first time can indeed feel overwhelming. The sheer volume of information and the complexity of herbal medicine may seem daunting at first glance.

However, the learning process becomes much more manageable and effective with the HERBS framework as your guide. This simple yet efficient framework breaks down herbal remedies into clear and digestible categories, making understanding their benefits and applications easier.

By following the HERBS framework, you can navigate the world of herbal medicine with confidence and clarity, empowering yourself to harness the healing power of herbs for your well-being.

- **H**: Healing immunity boosters are superheroes for your body's defense system. They contain powerful properties that fight inflammation, reduce swelling, and ease joint and muscle pain. Incorporating these herbs into your routine can boost your immune system, helping your body ward off illnesses and infections more effectively. Imagine feeling stronger and more resilient against common ailments like colds and the flu.
- **E**: Energizing adaptogens are natural energy boosters that help revitalize your body and mind. These herbs enhance your energy levels, giving you the vigor to tackle your day. They also improve blood circulation, ensuring oxygen and nutrients reach every body part efficiently. Picture yourself feeling more alert, focused, and ready to take on whatever challenges come your way.
- **R**: Respiratory soothers are a breath of fresh air for your lungs. They relieve respiratory issues ranging from the common cold to more severe conditions such as COPD. These herbs help to clear congestion, soothe irritated airways, and promote easier breathing. Imagine experiencing fewer coughing fits and breathing more freely, even during allergy season or times of illness.
- **B**: Brain boosters are like mental powerhouses that support cognitive function and brain health. Not only do they sharpen your focus and memory, but they also have the

potential to slow down the effects of conditions like dementia. These herbs nourish your brain cells, enhancing communication between neurons and supporting overall brain function. Envision yourself feeling sharper, more mentally alert, and maintaining cognitive vitality as you age.
- **S**: Stress relievers are natural soothers for the mind and body, offering a tranquil escape from the pressures of daily life. With their calming properties, they help alleviate tension, reduce anxiety, and promote relaxation. These herbs provide serenity, allowing you to unwind and find inner balance amid life's challenges.

This book also has a bonus chapter about other incredible natural remedies for skin care, fertility, pregnancy, hormonal balance, and children's medication. These complete the holistic healing approach.

WHAT YOU WILL GET OUT OF THIS BOOK

Discover the Power of Herbal Remedies is your ticket to:

Enhanced Well-Being

You will uncover a treasure trove of knowledge about herbal remedies that can transform your well-being. Imagine waking up each morning feeling refreshed, energized, and ready to seize the day, knowing that you have natural solutions to address any health concerns that may arise.

Improved Resilience

With the insights gained from this book, you'll develop a newfound sense of resilience against common ailments and health challenges. Picture yourself navigating through the seasons quickly as your body's immune system becomes stronger and more adept at warding off illnesses and infections.

Greater Vitality

As you incorporate the principles of herbal medicine into your daily life, you'll experience a surge in vitality and energy levels. Imagine having the stamina to pursue your passions, engage in physical activities, and spend quality time with loved ones without feeling drained or fatigued.

Mental Clarity

You'll notice a significant improvement in mental clarity and focus through the brain-boosting herbs and cognitive-enhancing remedies outlined in this book. Envision your mind becoming a wellspring of creativity and productivity, as you effortlessly tackle tasks and projects with precision and clarity.

Deeper Connection With Nature

Reading this book will enrich your understanding of herbal remedies and deepen your connection with the natural world. Picture yourself strolling through lush, green forests, breathing in the fresh scent of herbs and feeling a profound sense of harmony and balance with your environment.

PLEASE LET ME INTRODUCE MYSELF

I've walked the path of health struggles and triumphs. I've faced challenges just like you, navigating through health issues and seeking answers. With years of personal experience, research, and learning, I can genuinely say I have become an expert in herbal remedies.

But my journey wasn't always easy. I've experienced the frustrations of conventional medicine and the limitations it sometimes presents. Through trial and error, I have discovered the power of herbal remedies to alleviate my health concerns. This is why I understand firsthand the doubts and uncertainties of exploring alternative wellness approaches.

My passion for herbal medicine stems from my desire to share my knowledge and help others on their journey toward better health. I have dedicated myself to studying herbs, learning from experts, and honing my expertise. I can guide you through the intricacies of herbal remedies with compassion, understanding, and firsthand knowledge of their transformative influence on your well-being.

Before learning various herbal remedies, let us first highlight the amazing history of using herbs as medicine. We will also touch on the most common myths about herbal medicine and a short background of medicinal plants in pharmaceuticals. Let's meet in Chapter 1, where your journey begins!

THE TRUTH BEHIND THE HERBS

Long ago, our ancestors, lacking modern medicine, likely turned to plants for relief from pain and illness. While there are no written records, this likely marked the beginning of herbal medicine.

This chapter explores the history of herbal medicine, tracing its roots back to early humans. From ancient civilizations to indigenous cultures, herbs have played a vital role in healing. Discover the significance of herbal medicine throughout history, and learn how to find reliable herbal remedies and care for beginner-friendly herbs.

60,000 YEARS OF HERBAL USE

In prehistory, spanning over 60,000 years, humans began their relationship with herbal medicine. Despite no written records, our Paleolithic ancestors relied on plants for healing. Evidence from the Shanidar IV burial site in Iraq reveals pollen grains of medicinal plants alongside remains, hinting at intentional therapeutic use.

Mesopotamia - The Center of Early Herbal Remedy Use

In ancient Mesopotamia, the Sumerians were among the earliest civilizations to document herbal use. Cuneiform tablets from around 2600 BCE describe the cultivation and healing uses of herbs. These writings reflect the deep respect ancient cultures had for plant-based healing, shaping the course of herbal medicine across civilizations.

Herbal Therapy in Ancient Egypt

In Ancient Egypt, herbalism was integral to their advanced medical system. Documents like the Ebers and Edwin Smith Papyri list herbal remedies for different illnesses, including aloe vera, garlic, and juniper. Herbal medicine reflected their holistic view of health, blending with religious and cultural practices.

Herbal Use and Treatments in Ancient India

Ayurvedic medicine, from ancient India, is among the oldest holistic healing systems. It focuses on balancing mind, body, and spirit using herbal remedies like turmeric, ashwagandha, and holy basil. Texts like the *Charaka Samhita* and *Sushruta Samhita* detail the healing properties and uses of medicinal plants.

Herbal Treatments in China

Traditional Chinese Medicine (TCM) relies heavily on herbal medicine, which has been practiced for thousands of years. Herbal formulas, made from roots, leaves, and bark, are customized according to TCM principles. Classic texts like the *Shennong Ben Cao Jing* and the *Huangdi Neijing* provide detailed information on herbs to promote balance and wellness.

Hippocrates and Herbalism

Hippocrates, considered the father of Western medicine, highlighted the role of natural remedies in ancient Greece. He stressed the significance of diet, lifestyle, and herbs for health, famously saying, "Let food be thy medicine and medicine be thy food."

The Hippocratic Corpus, a collection of his medical texts, offers insights into plants' healing properties. His teachings paved the way for Western herbal medicine's development and its integration into modern healthcare.

Herbal Treatments During the Middle Ages

During the Middle Ages, herbalism thrived despite challenges. In Europe, monasteries were hubs of herbal knowledge, where monks grew medicinal plants and wrote herbal manuscripts. "Wise women" and "wise men" shared remedies in communities. Arabic medicine influenced European herbalism by translating Greek and Roman texts, enriching herbal traditions.

Despite suspicion, herbalism persisted, adapting to societal changes. Universities and guilds formalized herbal medicine, organizing plant knowledge. By the end of the Middle Ages, herbalism was firmly established in Europe and beyond, shaping modern herbal medicine.

MEDICINAL PLANTS IN PHARMACEUTICALS

Traditional medicine, often perceived as pre-scientific, continues to face skepticism despite its longstanding history and efficacy. However, it's remarkable to note that a significant portion, approximately 40%, of pharmaceutical products in use today are derived directly from plants.

Take the example of sweetwood and willow bark, which contain compounds with potent medicinal properties. Sweetwood, for instance, yields compounds used in cough syrups and expectorants, while willow bark serves as a natural source of salicin, the precursor to aspirin, a widely prescribed pain reliever.

These examples highlight the profound effect of traditional herbal knowledge on modern pharmaceuticals, challenging the notion that conventional medicine is outdated or inferior.

Widely Used Medications Derived from Plants and Herbs

Plants are crucial to many medications, providing over 100 active ingredients. For example, the purple foxglove yields compounds such as digitalin, digitoxin, and digoxin, used for heart conditions.

The opium poppy produces morphine for pain relief, while the Madagascar periwinkle provides vincristine and vinblastine for leukemia and lymphoma treatment. These examples highlight nature's role in pharmaceuticals, showing how plants drive medical progress.

Myths Surrounding Herbal Remedies

Let's focus on misconceptions about herbal medicine and shed some light on the truth behind them:

It's Neither Scientific nor Evidence-Based

Herbal medicine has a long history based on observation, tradition, and research. Though not all herbs undergo rigorous trials, many have been studied in labs and clinics, showing they are effective and safe for various health issues.

It's Expensive

Some herbal products can be expensive, but many are affordable and easy to find. You can grow some medicinal herbs at home or buy them inexpensively from local stores. Compared to conventional drugs, herbal medicine is often a more cost-effective option in the long term.

Herbalism and Homeopathy Are the Same

Herbalism and homeopathy both use natural substances for healing, but they have different approaches. Herbalism uses whole plants or extracts, while homeopathy uses highly diluted substances based on the principle of "like cures like." It's crucial to understand their differences and not confuse one with the other.

It's a Hippy Practice

Herbal medicine isn't limited to one group. It's been used by various cultures throughout history, from ancient times to today. Nowadays, it's becoming more accepted in mainstream healthcare globally, showing its effectiveness across different lifestyles and beliefs.

It's Just a Modern Fad

While herbal medicine may be experiencing a resurgence in popularity, its roots trace back thousands of years across diverse cultures worldwide. It's a persistent trend and a time-tested practice with deep historical and cultural significance.

Pharmaceuticals Are More Effective

Pharmaceutical drugs are important in healthcare, but herbal medicine offers a different approach with its own benefits. Herbal remedies can be effective depending on the person and the health issue, often complementing conventional treatments.

It's Natural, so It's Safe

Not all natural substances are safe. Herbs can interact with medications, have side effects, or be harmful if misused. Understanding the risks and benefits of herbal medicine is crucial for safe use.

WHAT TO LOOK FOR WHEN SOURCING HERBS

Practice care when sourcing herbs to ensure their quality, purity, and authenticity. Choosing reputable suppliers and understanding where your herbs come from helps you avoid potential contaminants or impurities, ensuring the safety and effectiveness of your herbal remedies. Remember these best practices.

- Exercise caution with herbal supplements due to potential interactions with conventional medications and strong effects; always consult your doctor before use.
- Educate yourself by seeking information from healthcare professionals and herbal supplement manufacturers to understand the herbs you're taking.

- Follow label instructions meticulously and adhere to prescribed dosages to minimize risks and maximize benefits.
- Consider consulting with a qualified herbalist or naturopathic doctor for personalized guidance and recommendations.
- Monitor for adverse reactions or side effects such as nausea, dizziness, headache, or upset stomach, and adjust dosage accordingly.
- Be vigilant for allergic reactions and seek immediate medical attention if symptoms such as trouble breathing occur.
- Choose herbal supplements from reputable manufacturers to ensure quality, effectiveness, and safety, recognizing that the source influences these factors significantly.

Prioritize organic materials in your herbal remedies for safety. Organic ingredients ensure your remedies are free from harmful chemicals like pesticides and herbicides, protecting your health.

Consider growing beginner-friendly medicinal plants at home. Cultivating your herbs lets you control growing conditions and ensure purity, enhancing your connection to nature's healing power.

Explore The Herbal Academy for guidance and resources on herbalism. Their website offers articles, courses, and community forums to support herbalists of all levels, enriching your herbal knowledge and practice.

QUICK TIPS TO START YOUR MEDICINAL HERB GARDEN

Starting a medicinal herb garden is rewarding and practical. It provides a sustainable source of organic remedies and saves money compared to buying from stores. Growing herbs organically guarantees pure, chemical-free ingredients for you and your family's health and well-being.

Many medicinal herbs also add flavor and nutrition to your meals, enriching your culinary experiences. Cultivate a diverse array of plants in your medicinal herb garden to enhance health and culinary delights.

Here's a step-by-step guide to help you grow culinary and medicinal herbs quickly:

1. **Create a list of common ailments**: Begin by identifying common health issues or ailments you and your family frequently encounter. This helps you prioritize which medicinal herbs to grow in your garden.
2. **Make a list of herbs you want to grow (after completing the HERBS framework)**: Refer to the HERBS framework to identify herbs that address the ailments on your list. Choose a variety of herbs with diverse medicinal properties to create a well-rounded herb garden.
3. **Plan when to start seeds**: Research the optimal time to start seeds for each herb based on your local climate and growing season. Some herbs may require an early start indoors, while others can be sown directly in the garden.
4. **Choosing the best location**: Select a location for your herb garden that receives adequate sunlight, typically 6-8 hours daily. Ensure the area is well-drained and protected from strong winds.

5. **Choosing the best soil**: Use well-draining, nutrient-rich soil for your herb garden. Consider amending the soil with compost or organic matter to improve its texture and fertility.
6. **Managing water and drainage**: Provide consistent moisture to your herbs by watering deeply and regularly, especially during hot and dry periods. Ensure proper drainage to prevent waterlogging, which can lead to root rot and other issues.
7. **Read the seed packet to know exactly what plants need**: Check the information provided on the seed packets for each herb to understand its specific growing requirements, including sunlight, soil, watering, and spacing. Follow the instructions carefully to ensure successful germination and growth.

By following these simple steps, you can create a thriving herb garden that enhances your culinary creations and provides natural remedies for common health concerns. Happy gardening!

CONCLUSION

After dipping our toes into the use of herbs for healing, it's time to get behind the science of medicinal plants and how they have so much potential. See you in the next chapter where we focus on the therapeutic effects of herbs. Let's go!

HOW YOUR HEALTH CAN BENEFIT FROM HERBAL REMEDIES

"Ounce for ounce, herbs and spices have more antioxidants than any other food group," declares Michael Greger. There is no doubt that a healthy, balanced diet is essential, but it's easy to forget the power spices hold! As you explore the world of herbal remedies and culinary delights, you'll uncover the profound effect that plants can have on your health and well-being, both physically and emotionally.

Imagine unlocking the potential of your spice rack not just to tantalize your taste buds but also to nourish your body and soul. In this chapter, you'll discover how plants improve health, not just through their nutritional value but also in a holistic sense. From ancient traditions to modern science, you'll gain a clear understanding of the transformative power of herbs and spices in enhancing your overall health and vitality.

PHYTOCHEMICALS KEEPING PLANTS HEALTHY

Phytochemicals are natural compounds in plants that help them stay healthy and protected from environmental stressors. These same phytochemicals offer numerous health benefits to humans when we consume plant-based foods, such as fruits, vegetables, herbs, and spices.

Incorporating phytochemical-rich foods into our diets can support our immune system, reduce inflammation, and lower the risk of chronic diseases, promoting overall health and well-being. Let's learn more about phytochemicals and their benefits to humans.

What Are Phytochemicals?

Phytochemicals are natural compounds found in plants, protecting them from stressors like UV radiation and pests. These compounds act as antioxidants, anti-inflammatories, and immune boosters for plants.

When humans consume phytochemical-rich foods like fruits, vegetables, legumes, herbs, and spices, we also benefit. Phytochemicals help reduce the risk of chronic diseases like cancer, heart disease, and diabetes. They support immune function, aid detoxification, and promote overall well-being.

Eating a variety of phytochemical-rich foods ensures we get diverse health benefits, helping us stay healthy and vibrant. Here are examples of herbs and plants that are rich in phytochemicals:

- **Turmeric**: It contains curcumin, a potent anti-inflammatory and antioxidant compound.
- **Garlic**: Rich in allicin, a compound with antimicrobial and heart-healthy properties.
- **Ginger**: Contains gingerol, known for its anti-inflammatory and digestive benefits.
- **Green tea**: Loaded with catechins, powerful antioxidants that promote heart health and metabolism.
- **Berries**: Packed with anthocyanins, flavonoids, and polyphenols that support brain health and reduce inflammation.
- **Cruciferous vegetables**: Contain sulforaphane and glucosinolates, compounds with anti-cancer properties.
- **Cinnamon**: Rich in cinnamaldehyde, known for its anti-inflammatory and blood sugar-regulating effects.
- **Rosemary**: Contains rosmarinic acid and carnosic acid, potent antioxidants with neuroprotective properties.
- **Flaxseeds**: High in lignans, omega-3 fatty acids, and fiber, which support heart health and digestive function.
- **Spinach**: Contains lutein, zeaxanthin, and chlorophyll, compounds that promote eye health and provide antioxidant protection.

Phytochemicals in Boosting Immune System Health

Phytochemicals boost the immune system by fighting infections and diseases with their antioxidant, anti-inflammatory, and antimicrobial properties. Adding phytochemical-rich foods to our diets enhances resilience and overall well-being. Here are examples of phytochemical-rich foods that support immune system health:

- **Elderberries**: Rich in flavonoids and anthocyanins, elderberries possess potent antiviral properties and can help alleviate symptoms of colds and the flu.
- **Garlic**: Contains allicin, a compound with antimicrobial properties that can help fend off infections and support immune function.
- **Ginger**: Loaded with gingerol and other bioactive compounds, ginger exhibits anti-inflammatory and antioxidant effects, contributing to immune system resilience.
- **Turmeric**: Contains curcumin, a potent anti-inflammatory and antioxidant compound that supports immune function and overall health.
- **Citrus fruits**: Packed with vitamin C and flavonoids, citrus fruits such as oranges, lemons, and grapefruits help boost immune system function and protect against infections.

Phytochemicals in Cancer Prevention

Phytochemicals prevent cancer by protecting cells from damage and inhibiting cancer growth (Bramlet, 2017). They act as antioxidants, neutralizing harmful free radicals, and have anti-inflammatory properties that reduce chronic inflammation linked to cancer.

Adding phytochemical-rich foods to our diets lowers cancer risk and boosts overall health. Here are examples of phytochemical-rich foods known for their cancer-preventive properties:

- **Cruciferous vegetables**: Contain glucosinolates and sulforaphane, which inhibit the growth of cancer cells and promote detoxification processes.

- **Berries**: Rich in anthocyanins, flavonoids, and ellagic acid, with antioxidant and anti-inflammatory effects that may help prevent cancer development.
- **Tomatoes**: They contain lycopene, a carotenoid with potent antioxidant properties that may help reduce the risk of prostate, breast, lung, and stomach cancers.
- **Green tea**: Contains catechins, particularly epigallocatechin gallate (EGCG), which has been studied for its potential to inhibit cancer cell growth and induce apoptosis, or cell death (Bing-Huei, 2020).
- **Turmeric**: Contains curcumin, a compound with powerful anti-inflammatory and antioxidant effects that may help prevent cancer by inhibiting the growth of tumor cells and reducing inflammation in the body.

Phytochemicals for Brain Health

Phytochemicals aid brain health by protecting against cognitive decline and neurodegenerative diseases (Davinelli, 2016). They fight oxidative stress and inflammation in the brain, crucial factors in cognitive decline.

Foods rich in phytochemicals improve memory, focus, and brain function by fostering new brain cell growth and safeguarding existing neurons from harm. Here are examples of phytochemical-rich foods known for their brain-boosting properties:

- **Blueberries**: Rich in anthocyanins and flavonoids, blueberries have been shown to improve memory and cognitive function, as well as reduce the risk of age-related cognitive decline.

- **Walnuts**: Packed with omega-3 fatty acids, antioxidants, and polyphenols, walnuts support brain health by improving cognitive function and reducing inflammation in the brain.
- **Dark chocolate**: Contains flavonoids and antioxidants that enhance blood flow to the brain, improve cognitive function, and protect against age-related cognitive decline.
- **Leafy greens (e.g., spinach, kale, Swiss chard)**: High in vitamins, minerals, and phytochemicals such as lutein and zeaxanthin, leafy greens support brain health by reducing inflammation and oxidative stress and promoting neuroplasticity.
- **Turmeric**: Contains curcumin, a compound with potent anti-inflammatory and antioxidant properties that may help improve memory, reduce the risk of Alzheimer's disease, and protect against age-related cognitive decline.

Phytochemicals for a Healthy Heart

Phytochemicals support heart health by reducing inflammation, enhancing blood vessel function, and lowering cholesterol levels. They're present in plant-based foods and aid in preventing cardiovascular diseases.

These foods also offer antioxidants that shield against oxidative stress, a factor in heart disease. Adding them to your diet can lower blood pressure, enhance circulation, and lower the risk of heart attacks and strokes. Here are examples of phytochemical-rich foods known for their heart-healthy properties:

- **Oats**: Rich in beta-glucans, oats help lower cholesterol levels and improve heart health by reducing the risk of coronary artery disease.

- **Berries**: Loaded with anthocyanins, flavonoids, and polyphenols, berries help lower blood pressure, improve blood vessel function, and reduce inflammation, promoting heart health.
- **Fatty fish (e.g., salmon, mackerel, sardines)**: High in omega-3 fatty acids, fatty fish help reduce triglyceride levels, lower blood pressure, and prevent blood clots, reducing the risk of heart disease and stroke.
- **Legumes (e.g., lentils, chickpeas, beans)**: Packed with soluble fiber, legumes help lower cholesterol levels, stabilize blood sugar levels, and reduce the risk of heart disease.
- **Dark chocolate**: Contains flavonoids that improve blood flow to the heart, lower blood pressure, and reduce the risk of heart disease when consumed in moderation.

CONCLUSION

Now that the theory behind herbal remedies is clear, the next step is learning simple techniques to make herbal remedies. We will learn how to make teas, infusions, decoctions, tinctures, syrups, salves, poultices, and compresses. This is a chapter worth waiting for! See you in Chapter 3.

MAKING YOUR HERBAL REMEDIES

Part of harnessing the power of herbs is learning to be confident in crafting various remedies. In this chapter, you'll learn how to concoct different herbal remedies and increase your confidence.

As you explore the different ways to make teas, infusions, decoctions, and tinctures, you might notice that we don't include exact measurements in our recipes. That's because we respect the uniqueness of each individual. For example, if you love chili, you might add more spice than someone trying it for the first time.

The amounts you use will also depend on whether your ingredients are fresh or dry. Don't worry; we'll guide you with general ratios for each remedy, giving you the confidence to experiment and find what works best for you.

MAKING TEAS AND INFUSIONS

Herbal teas and infusions are both beverages made by steeping herbs in hot water, but they differ in their steeping time and strength.

Herbal Teas

Herbal teas are made by steeping herbs in hot water for a short period, usually around 5-10 minutes. This gentle steeping process extracts the flavors and some of the medicinal properties of the herbs, resulting in a light and refreshing beverage.

Infusions

Infusions require steeping herbs in hot water for 15-30 minutes or more, drawing out potent medicinal compounds and flavors.

Herbal teas and infusions offer health benefits like relaxation, digestion aid, and immune support, depending on the herbs. They're appreciated for both their medicinal effects and delightful tastes, providing soothing qualities.

How to Make Infusions and Teas

Brewing herbal teas and infusions lets you experience herbs' medicinal benefits. For tea, steep herbs briefly, strain, and enjoy a delicate flavor with mild effects. Infusions yield a stronger taste.

Choose between teas and infusions based on your taste preference and desired strength. Enjoy the process and the wonderful flavors they bring!

Examples of Teas and Infusions

- **Chamomile Tea**: Known for its calming properties, chamomile tea is made from the dried flowers of the chamomile plant and is often consumed before bedtime to promote relaxation and better sleep.
- **Peppermint Infusion**: Peppermint infusion is made from the leaves of the peppermint plant. It's refreshing and commonly used to aid digestion, soothe upset stomachs, and relieve headaches.
- **Ginger Tea**: Made from fresh or dried ginger root, ginger tea is renowned for its spicy and warming flavor. It alleviates nausea, reduces inflammation, and boosts the immune system.
- **Lemon Balm Infusion**: Lemon balm infusion is made from the leaves of the lemon balm plant. It has a mild lemony flavor and is frequently enjoyed for its calming effects, reducing anxiety and promoting relaxation.
- **Green Tea**: Green tea is made from the leaves of the Camellia sinensis plant and is known for its antioxidant properties. It improves brain function, helps with fat loss, and reduces the risk of certain diseases.

WHEN A DECOCTION IS NEEDED

An herbal decoction is a potent herbal remedy made by boiling tough plant parts like roots or seeds in water for a long time. Unlike teas, decoctions need extended heating to draw out medicinal properties from hard plant materials.

This method extracts therapeutic compounds that other techniques may miss. Decoctions suit herbs with sturdy textures or those with active components not easily soluble in water.

After preparation, strain and consume the decoction hot or cold, depending on preference. Traditional herbal medicine often relies on decoctions to treat digestive and respiratory problems.

Qualities of a Good Decoction

Ayurvedic medicine is a holistic healing system that originated in ancient India over 3,000 years ago. It emphasizes balance between the body, mind, and spirit through herbal remedies, dietary adjustments, yoga, and meditation to promote overall health and well-being. Ayurvedic medicine states the qualities of an excellent decoction to maximize its therapeutic benefits.

- **Potency**: A good decoction should be potent, meaning it contains a concentrated amount of active constituents for effective medicinal effects.
- **Balanced Doshas**: Ayurvedic decoctions aim to balance the doshas, fundamental energies governing bodily functions, promoting equilibrium.
- **Digestibility**: Herbs chosen for the decoction should match the individual's digestive capacity to prevent adverse effects.
- **Correct Preparation**: Ayurvedic texts guide the proper selection of herbs and cooking methods to extract maximum medicinal properties.
- **Taste**: A balanced taste profile incorporating sweet, sour, salty, bitter, pungent, and astringent tastes enhances therapeutic effects.
- **Safety**: Ayurvedic decoctions must be made from high-quality, organic herbs, ensuring safety and efficacy, free from impurities.

By adhering to these qualities, decoctions can effectively promote health and well-being while addressing specific imbalances or ailments in the body.

Examples of Decoctions

- **Ashwagandha Decoction**: Made from the roots of the ashwagandha plant, this decoction is valued in Ayurvedic medicine for its adaptogenic properties, helping to combat stress and promote vitality.
- **Cinnamon Decoction**: Prepared from cinnamon bark, this decoction is often used to regulate blood sugar levels, improve digestion, and relieve menstrual discomfort.
- **Licorice Decoction**: Made from licorice root, this decoction is known for its soothing effects on the throat and respiratory system, making it useful for coughs, colds, and sore throats.
- **Dandelion Root Decoction**: Utilizing the roots of the dandelion plant, this decoction is prized for its diuretic properties, promoting kidney health and aiding in detoxification.
- **Triphala Decoction**: Comprising a blend of three fruits—amla, bibhitaki, and haritaki—Triphala decoction is revered in Ayurveda for its cleansing and rejuvenating effects on the digestive system, supporting regularity and overall wellness.

TINCTURES FOR ADDITIONAL POTENCY

Tinctures are potent herbal extracts made by soaking herbs in alcohol to draw out their medicinal compounds. After a few weeks or months, the liquid is strained, leaving behind a concentrated herbal solution.

Tinctures have a long shelf life and are easy to use. They can be taken orally by adding a few drops to water or applied topically for relief. Tinctures are favored by those seeking potent and convenient remedies because of their concentrated herbal doses.

Using the Right Alcohol in Making Tinctures

Choosing the correct alcohol is key for effective tinctures. The Fold Method matches alcohol strength to the plant's water content, optimizing extraction. Using the right herb-to-alcohol ratio ensures potency. These steps ensure high-quality tinctures with desired health benefits.

Examples of Tinctures

- **Echinacea Tincture**: Extracted from the echinacea plant, this tincture is commonly used to boost the immune system and shorten the duration of colds and the flu.
- **Valerian Tincture**: Derived from the root of the valerian plant, this tincture is prized for its soothing properties, helping to promote relaxation and improve sleep quality.
- **St. John's Wort Tincture**: Made from the flowering tops of the St. John's wort plant, this tincture is often used to alleviate symptoms of mild to moderate depression and anxiety.
- **Milk Thistle Tincture**: Extracted from the seeds of the milk thistle plant, this tincture supports liver health and aids in detoxification by promoting the regeneration of liver cells.
- **Hawthorn Berry Tincture**: Derived from the berries of the hawthorn tree, this tincture is known for its cardiovascular benefits, including improving circulation, lowering blood pressure, and supporting heart health.

MAKING HERBAL SYRUPS

Herbal syrups offer sweet ways to benefit from herbs' medicinal properties. Made with natural ingredients like honey or sugar, they're easy to consume. Popular for soothing coughs and sore throats, they provide relief while delivering herbal benefits.

How to Make Simple Herbal Syrups

1. **Choose Your Herbs**: Select the herbs you want to use based on their medicinal properties and flavors. Popular choices include elderberry for immune support, ginger for digestion, and lemon balm for relaxation.
2. **Prepare the Herbs**: Wash them thoroughly and chop them into smaller pieces to release their flavors and medicinal compounds.
3. **Create an Infusion**: Place the chopped herbs in a saucepan and cover them with water. Simmer the mixture over low heat for about 20-30 minutes to create a strong herbal infusion.
4. **Strain the Liquid**: Once the infusion is ready, strain the liquid through a fine mesh sieve or cheesecloth to remove the solid herb particles.
5. **Add Sweetener**: Return the strained liquid to the saucepan and add your sweeteners, such as honey, maple syrup, or sugar. Stir until the sweetener is completely dissolved.
6. **Simmer and Thicken**: Continue simmering the mixture over low heat until it thickens to the desired syrup consistency. This may take about 20-30 minutes.
7. **Cool and Store:** Once the syrup has thickened, remove it from the heat and allow it to cool completely. Transfer the syrup to clean, sterilized bottles or jars for storage.

8. **Enjoy Your Herbal Syrup**: Use your homemade herbal syrup as a delicious topping for pancakes, waffles, or desserts. Mix it with hot water to create a soothing herbal tea, or add it to smoothies to boost flavor and nutrition.

Once the herbal decoction is ready, it can be easily transformed into syrup by adding sugar or honey, with honey being the preferred choice due to its health benefits. Adding sugar or honey helps sweeten the decoction, making it more palatable and enjoyable while preserving its medicinal properties.

Making herbal syrups at home is a fun and rewarding way to incorporate the healing properties of herbs into your daily routine. Experiment with different herbs and sweeteners to create unique syrups that suit your taste preferences and health needs.

Examples of Herbal Syrups

- **Elderberry Syrup**: Made from the berries of the elder tree, elderberry syrup is rich in antioxidants and is often used to boost the immune system and shorten the duration of colds and the flu.
- **Marshmallow Root Syrup**: Derived from the root of the marshmallow plant, this syrup has soothing properties that can help relieve coughs, sore throats, and digestive discomfort.
- **Mullein Syrup**: Prepared from the leaves and flowers of the mullein plant, this syrup is prized for its expectorant qualities, making it useful for loosening mucus and easing respiratory congestion.
- **Thyme Syrup**: Thyme syrup is made from the leaves of the thyme herb and is known for its antimicrobial

properties, which can help fight bacterial infections and support respiratory health.
- **Ginger Syrup**: Ginger syrup, crafted from ginger root, is revered for its anti-inflammatory and digestive benefits. It can ease nausea, soothe upset stomachs, and add a spicy, warming flavor to beverages and recipes.

Oil and Vinegar Infusions

In herbal remedies, oil and vinegar infusions are preparations where medicinal herbs or plants are steeped in either oil or vinegar to extract their beneficial properties.

Oil and vinegar infusions are simple methods to extract herbal benefits.

- Oil infusions involve soaking herbs in carrier oils, creating potent remedies for skin issues and muscle tension relief.
- Vinegar infusions use apple cider vinegar to draw out herbal properties, offering internal tonics or external disinfectants.

Both infusions are versatile, serving in salves, liniments, and baths, addressing diverse health needs naturally.

How to Make Oil and Vinegar Infusions

In herbal remedies, oil and vinegar infusions can be made using the following methods:

Hot Method for Oil Infusions

In the hot method, herbs are heated with oil to speed up infusion. Heat gently warms the oil and herbs together, helping the oil absorb the herbs' benefits faster. After straining, the infused oil is ready for use in remedies.

Cold Method for Oil Infusions

The cold method involves letting herbs steep in oil at room temperature for an extended period, usually a few weeks. This gentler approach allows the oil to slowly absorb the herbal benefits. After the steeping period, strain the oil, producing a potent herbal-infused oil.

Cold Method for Vinegar Infusions

For herbal vinegar infusions, the cold method is commonly used. Herbs are submerged in vinegar and steeped at room temperature for several weeks. This slow infusion process allows the vinegar to absorb the medicinal properties of the herbs. After straining, the infused vinegar is suitable for internal or external use.

Choosing a versatile oil that can be used both for cooking and topically, like olive oil, saves money and allows for a dual-purpose herbal remedy. This approach offers a practical and cost-effective way to incorporate herbal infusions into culinary and medicinal practices.

SALVES FOR TOPICAL USE

Salves are herbal blends mixed with bases like beeswax, oil, or fat, forming semisolid preparations. Applied on the skin, they deliver herbs' benefits directly, easing irritation, aiding wound healing, and reducing inflammation.

Ingredients vary based on the herbs' properties and intended use, targeting inflammation, infection, pain, or skin soothing. Salves are convenient, versatile remedies for skin issues, made by infusing oils with herbs.

How to Make Salves

1. **Gather Your Ingredients**: You'll need infused herbal oil, beeswax, and any additional essential oils or herbs you want to include for added benefits or fragrance.
2. **Prepare Your Work Area**: Set up a clean, dry work area and gather your equipment, including a double boiler or heatproof bowl, stirring utensils, and containers for your salve.
3. **Melt the Beeswax**: Melt the beeswax over low heat in a double boiler or heatproof bowl. The amount of beeswax you use will determine the consistency of your salve — more beeswax creates a firmer salve, while less beeswax results in a softer consistency.
4. **Add the Infused Oil**: Once the beeswax is melted, gradually add your infused herbal oil, stirring gently to combine. Adjust the ratio of oil to beeswax as needed to achieve your desired consistency.
5. **Optional Additions**: If desired, add a few drops of essential oils for fragrance or additional therapeutic benefits. Stir well to incorporate.

6. **Pour Into Containers**: Carefully pour the liquid salve mixture into clean, dry containers, such as jars or tins, before solidifying. Leave the containers open until the salve has cooled and solidified completely.
7. **Label and Store**: Once the salve has cooled and solidified, label your containers with the date and ingredients used. Store the salves in a cool, dry place away from direct sunlight.

Examples of Salves

- **Calendula Salve**: Made from calendula flowers, this salve is renowned for its soothing and healing properties and is often used to treat minor cuts, burns, and skin irritations.
- **Arnica Salve**: Derived from the arnica plant, this is valued for its anti-inflammatory effects, making it popular for relieving muscle aches, bruises, and sprains.
- **Comfrey Salve**: Comfrey salve is from the comfrey plant and is prized for its ability to promote skin regeneration and reduce inflammation, making it beneficial for wounds, cuts, and eczema.
- **Lavender Salve**: A salve infused with lavender flowers, cherished for its calming aroma and skin-soothing properties, is often used to alleviate minor burns, insect bites, and dry skin.
- **Tea Tree Salve**: Tea tree salve contains tea tree oil and is known for its antiseptic and antimicrobial properties, effectively treating acne, minor cuts, and fungal infections.

POULTICES AND COMPRESSES

Poultices and compresses are traditional herbal remedies used externally to alleviate pain, reduce inflammation, promote healing, and relieve various ailments.

Poultices

Poultices are herbal mixtures applied on the skin. Made by blending herbs with hot water, they form a paste. Spread on cloth or skin, they're covered to stay in place.

Compresses

Compresses are like poultices. A cloth is soaked in herbal liquid, hot or cold, then applied to the skin after wringing.

How to Make a Poultice

Making a poultice out of fresh herbs is a simple process. Here's how you can do it:

1. **Choose Your Herbs**: Select fresh herbs that possess medicinal properties suitable for your intended use. Common herbs used in poultices include plantain, comfrey, calendula, chamomile, and peppermint.
2. **Prepare the Herbs**: Wash the fresh herbs thoroughly under running water to remove dirt or debris. Pat them dry with a clean towel.
3. **Crush or Chop the Herbs**: Using a mortar and pestle, food processor, or simply chopping with a knife, crush or chop the fresh herbs to release their juices and activate their

medicinal properties. You want to break down the herbs to a coarse consistency.
4. **Apply the Herbs**: Place the crushed or chopped herbs directly onto the affected skin area. You can also spread them onto a clean cloth or gauze to create a poultice that can be applied more efficiently.
5. **Cover the Poultice**: Once the herbs are applied, cover the area with a clean cloth or bandage to hold the poultice in place.

Fresh herb poultices relieve inflammation, soothe minor wounds or burns, reduce swelling, and promote skin healing. They offer a natural and effective way to harness the healing properties of fresh herbs for topical applications.

How to Make a Compress

To make a compress, follow these simple steps.

1. **Prepare the Decoction**: Start by brewing a decoction using medicinal herbs of your choice. Allow the decoction to cool to a comfortable temperature.
2. **Select Your Cloth**: Choose a clean, soft cloth that is large enough to cover the affected body area. Natural fabrics like cotton or linen work well for making compresses.
3. **Dip the Cloth**: Once the decoction has cooled, dip the cloth into the liquid, ensuring it is fully saturated but not dripping excessively. You want the fabric to absorb enough herbal solution to provide effective treatment.
4. **Wring Out Excess Liquid**: Gently wring out the cloth to remove any excess liquid. You want the compress to be moist but not dripping wet.

5. **Apply to the Affected Area**: Place the moistened cloth onto the affected body area. Make sure the compress covers the area thoroughly.
6. **Secure in Place**: Use medical tape or a bandage, or simply hold the compress in place with your hand to ensure it stays in position.
7. **Leave in Place**: Allow the compress to remain on the affected area for about 20-30 minutes, as recommended by your herbalist or healthcare provider.

Compresses can be used for various purposes, including reducing inflammation, soothing sore muscles, relieving headaches, and promoting relaxation. They offer a gentle and effective way to deliver the healing properties of medicinal herbs directly to the skin.

Examples of Compresses and Poultices

- **Warm Ginger Compress**: A cloth soaked in warm ginger-infused water, applied to the affected area to ease muscle soreness, improve circulation, and reduce inflammation.
- **Mustard Poultice**: Ground mustard seeds mixed with water and applied to the chest to alleviate congestion, relieve coughs, and promote respiratory health.
- **Epsom Salt Compress**: A cloth soaked in warm water mixed with Epsom salt, placed on sore muscles or bruises to reduce pain and inflammation and promote relaxation.
- **Chamomile Poultice**: Crushed chamomile flowers mixed with hot water are applied to the skin to soothe irritation, reduce redness, and promote healing, especially for minor skin inflammations.

- **Turmeric Compress**: Turmeric powder mixed with warm water, applied to joints or bruises to reduce pain and inflammation and support healing. It is known for its anti-inflammatory properties.

CONCLUSION

Now that know all the methods to make herbal remedies, it's time to decide which medicinal plants are going to bring the best benefits. Chapter 4 highlights Healing Immunity Boosters, the first letter in the HERBS framework. These herbs boost the immune system, ease inflammation, and much more. It's time for H in Chapter 4.

H: HEALING IMMUNITY BOOSTERS

In this chapter, we'll focus on one of the most hardworking systems of the human body: our immune system. We'll highlight how the immune system works, why it is linked to inflammation, and how herbal remedies can improve immune system health and ease inflammation.

We'll explore how certain herbs and spices possess remarkable anti-inflammatory properties that can help combat inflammation and support your health. Through simple recipes and insights, you'll learn how to harness the healing power of these natural remedies to promote wellness and vitality in your daily life.

So, let's start our journey to discover the wonders of anti-inflammatory herbs and spices, help nurture your body, and enhance your overall well-being.

HOW IS THE IMMUNE SYSTEM LINKED TO INFLAMMATION?

When the immune system is activated, it mobilizes a complex network of cells, tissues, and molecules to defend the body against harmful invaders such as bacteria, viruses, and other pathogens.

This activation triggers a cascade of events aimed at identifying and neutralizing the threat to maintain the body's health and integrity. Here's what happens when the immune system is activated:

- **Recognition of Pathogens**: Specialized cells in the immune system, such as macrophages and dendritic cells, detect the presence of pathogens by recognizing specific molecules known as antigens on their surface.
- **Activation of Immune Response**: Upon detection of pathogens, the immune system initiates an immune response. This involves the production and release of cytokine signaling molecules, which serve as messengers to coordinate the immune response.
- **Recruitment of Immune Cells**: Cytokines signal the recruitment of various immune cells, including white blood cells such as neutrophils, T cells, and B cells to the site of infection or inflammation.
- **Elimination of Pathogens**: Immune cells work together to neutralize and eliminate the invading pathogens. This process may involve phagocytosis, where immune cells engulf and digest pathogens, and the production of antibodies to target specific pathogens for destruction.
- **Inflammatory Response**: Inflammation is a critical component of the immune response. It is characterized by redness, swelling, heat, and pain at the site of infection or

injury. Inflammation helps to isolate and contain the infection, as well as promote tissue repair and healing.

The immune system's activation and inflammatory response protect the body against infections and maintain health and well-being. However, dysregulation or overactivation of the immune system leads to chronic inflammation and contributes to various health conditions, including autoimmune diseases, allergies, and chronic inflammatory disorders.

Understanding the intricate relationship between the immune system and inflammation is crucial for maintaining optimal health and supporting immune function.

Acute vs. Chronic Inflammation

Acute inflammation is a short-term, localized response of the body's immune system to injury, infection, or tissue damage. It is characterized by the classic signs of inflammation, including redness, swelling, heat, and pain. It is typically resolved within a few days to weeks as the underlying cause is addressed and the affected tissues heal.

Chronic inflammation, on the other hand, is a prolonged and persistent inflammatory response that lasts over an extended period, often months to years. Unlike acute inflammation, chronic inflammation may occur silently without the classic signs of acute inflammation.

This type of inflammation can be triggered by a variety of factors, including unresolved infections, autoimmune disorders, prolonged exposure to environmental toxins, unhealthy lifestyle habits, and underlying medical conditions.

Common Conditions Associated With Inflammation

You might be experiencing common inflammation-related conditions, such as arthritis or allergies. Understanding these conditions can help you manage symptoms and improve your well-being.

- **Arthritis**: Both rheumatoid arthritis and osteoarthritis involve inflammation of the joints, leading to pain, stiffness, and reduced mobility.
- **Cardiovascular Diseases**: Chronic inflammation plays a crucial role in the development and progression of conditions such as atherosclerosis, heart disease, and stroke.
- **Allergies and Asthma**: Inflammatory responses in the respiratory system contribute to the symptoms of allergies and asthma, including wheezing, coughing, and shortness of breath.
- **Inflammatory Bowel Diseases (IBD)**: Conditions such as Crohn's disease and ulcerative colitis involve chronic inflammation of the digestive tract, leading to abdominal pain, diarrhea, and other gastrointestinal symptoms.
- **Diabetes**: Inflammation is involved in insulin resistance and the development of type 2 diabetes, as well as diabetic complications such as neuropathy and cardiovascular disease.
- **Skin Conditions**: Inflammatory skin disorders such as psoriasis, eczema, and acne are characterized by skin inflammation, leading to redness, itching, and irritation.
- **Neurological Disorders**: Chronic inflammation has been linked to neurodegenerative diseases such as Alzheimer's disease, Parkinson's disease, and multiple sclerosis.

Understanding the distinction between acute and chronic inflammation and recognizing the associated conditions is essential for identifying potential health risks and implementing strategies to support immune health and reduce inflammation in the body.

BEST PLANTS WITH HEALING IMMUNITY BOOSTERS

In anti-inflammatory relief, exploring natural options can prove beneficial in managing discomfort and enhancing overall wellness. Experimenting with therapeutic plants may provide natural relief from inflammation, contributing positively to your health and well-being. Here are the top anti-inflammatory plants for you.

Turmeric

Turmeric is a vibrant yellow spice originating from the Curcuma longa plant, common in South Asia. It boasts anti-inflammatory properties attributed to curcumin, its active compound. Curcumin moderates inflammatory pathways, reducing pro-inflammatory molecule production and easing inflammation.

To use turmeric's anti-inflammatory benefits, you can try:

1. **Turmeric Tea**: Brew a cup by adding a teaspoon of ground turmeric to hot water or milk, enhancing taste and absorption with a dash of black pepper and honey.
2. **Golden Milk**: Blend turmeric with warm milk, cinnamon, ginger, and sweeteners like honey or maple syrup for a comforting drink.
3. **Turmeric Smoothies**: Integrate a teaspoon of turmeric into daily smoothies along with fruits, greens, and healthy fats such as avocado or coconut oil.

4. **Curries and Stir-Fries**: Use turmeric generously in dishes like curries, soups, stews, and stir-fries to add flavor, color, and anti-inflammatory properties, complementing it with spices like ginger, garlic, cumin, and coriander.
5. **Turmeric Supplements**: Consider turmeric supplements or capsules containing standardized curcumin extracts for a concentrated dose of anti-inflammatory compounds, with guidance from a healthcare professional regarding dosage and suitability.

Ginger

Ginger, originating from Southeast Asia, is valued for its rhizome used in both cuisine and traditional medicine. Its intense, spicy flavor with a hint of sweetness makes it versatile.

Ginger's anti-inflammatory properties stem from bioactive compounds like gingerol, shogaol, and paradol, which inhibit inflammatory molecule production, easing conditions such as arthritis, muscle soreness, and digestive issues.

To harness ginger's anti-inflammatory effects, use:

1. **Ginger Tea**: Slice fresh ginger root and steep in hot water. Enhance flavor with lemon juice and honey.
2. **Ginger Shots**: Blend fresh ginger with water or juice, then strain for a potent tonic to start the day and boost immunity.
3. **Ginger Infusions**: Add grated ginger to soups, stews, and broths for flavor and anti-inflammatory benefits.
4. **Ginger Supplements**: Consider ginger capsules or extracts for concentrated anti-inflammatory compounds, beneficial for chronic inflammatory conditions.

5. **Ginger in Cooking**: Incorporate ginger into stir-fries, sauces, marinades, and dressings to add zest and aroma, complementing various cuisines.

Rosemary

Rosemary, an aromatic evergreen herb from the Mediterranean and part of the mint family, is known for its fragrant aroma and diverse uses in culinary dishes, herbal remedies, and aromatherapy.

Its anti-inflammatory properties are attributed to bioactive compounds like rosmarinic acid, carnosol, and caffeic acid. These compounds inhibit pro-inflammatory enzymes and molecules, easing conditions such as arthritis, muscle soreness, and respiratory issues.

To harness rosemary's anti-inflammatory effects, try:

1. **Rosemary Infusion**: Steep fresh or dried rosemary leaves in hot water for a fragrant herbal tea, alone or combined with herbs like mint or lemon balm.
2. **Rosemary Oil**: Infuse fresh rosemary leaves in carrier oils like olive or coconut oil for topical use in massaging sore muscles, joints, or adding to bathwater for a luxurious experience.
3. **Culinary Use**: Add rosemary to roasted vegetables, meat dishes, soups, and sauces for its robust flavor and pine-like aroma, enhancing taste and nutritional value.
4. **Aromatherapy**: Diffuse rosemary essential oil to create a stimulating atmosphere promoting mental clarity, concentration, emotional well-being, and respiratory support.

5. **Herbal Remedies**: Explore traditional formulations incorporating rosemary in herbal tinctures, salves, compresses, and poultices to address inflammatory conditions and promote overall health.

Borage

Borage, or Borago officinalis, is an annual herb native to the Mediterranean but grown worldwide, known for its vibrant blue star-shaped flowers and cucumber-flavored, hairy leaves. It's prized for both ornamental beauty and potential medicinal benefits.

Its anti-inflammatory properties come from gamma-linolenic acid (GLA), an omega-6 fatty acid. GLA modulates the body's inflammatory response, reducing pro-inflammatory molecules while enhancing anti-inflammatory compounds. This makes borage potentially beneficial for conditions like arthritis, eczema, and respiratory issues.

To harness borage's anti-inflammatory effects, use:

1. **Borage Tea**: Steep fresh or dried borage leaves and flowers in hot water for a refreshing herbal beverage, hot or cold.
2. **Borage Oil**: Extracted from borage seeds, rich in GLA and other fatty acids. It can be taken orally as a supplement or applied topically to soothe inflammation and promote skin health.
3. **Culinary Use**: Add fresh borage leaves and flowers to salads, soups, sauces, and garnishes for color, flavor, and nutrition, complementing various dishes.
4. **Herbal Remedies**: Explore traditional formulations like tinctures, extracts, and topicals that include borage to

reduce inflammation, boost immunity, and enhance vitality.
5. **Supplements**: Consider borage oil supplements or GLA capsules to support your diet and body's natural anti-inflammatory pathways, with guidance from a healthcare professional regarding dosage and usage.

Devil's Claw

Devil's claw, or Harpagophytum procumbens, hails from southern Africa and earns its name from its fruit's claw-like appearance. Traditionally utilized in African medicine, devil's claw is renowned globally for its potential health advantages.

Its anti-inflammatory prowess comes from compounds like harpagoside and harpagide, which deter inflammatory enzyme and molecule production, thereby reducing inflammation and alleviating pain linked to arthritis, rheumatism, and muscle soreness.

To use devil's claw's anti-inflammatory benefits, try:

1. **Herbal Tea**: Steep dried devil's claw root in hot water for a soothing tea, consuming up to three times daily to mitigate inflammation and bolster joint health.
2. **Tinctures and Extracts**: Opt for devil's claw tinctures or liquid extracts, concentrated forms of the plant's active compounds. Follow dosage instructions on the product label or seek guidance from a healthcare professional.
3. **Topical Applications**: Apply devil's claw gel or cream directly to the affected area to diminish inflammation and ease pain associated with arthritis, tendonitis, and other inflammatory conditions. Massage gently until absorbed.
4. **Capsules and Tablets**: Access devil's claw in capsule or tablet format for convenient ingestion. Adhere to

recommended dosages mentioned on the product packaging or as advised by a healthcare practitioner.

Before using devil's claw, consult a healthcare provider, especially if you have existing health conditions, are pregnant or breastfeeding, or are taking medications that may interact with the herb.

Stinging Nettle

Stinging nettle, or Urtica dioica, is a perennial plant found across Europe, Asia, Africa, and North America, recognized by its serrated leaves and stinging hairs. Despite its prickly nature, stinging nettle has been valued for centuries for its medicinal and culinary applications.

Its anti-inflammatory properties come from bioactive compounds like flavonoids, phenolic acids, and lignans. These components hinder the production of inflammatory cytokines and enzymes, making stinging nettle effective against conditions such as arthritis, allergies, and skin inflammation.

To utilize stinging nettle's anti-inflammatory benefits, use:

1. **Herbal Tea**: Steep dried stinging nettle leaves in hot water for a nourishing beverage, consuming it up to three times daily to alleviate inflammation and enhance overall health.
2. **Cooked Greens**: Incorporate fresh or cooked stinging nettle leaves into various dishes like soups, stews, omelets, and pasta for added nutrition and flavor.
3. **Capsules and Extracts**: Opt for stinging nettle supplements in capsule or liquid extract form for a concentrated dose of anti-inflammatory compounds, following recommended dosages or seeking guidance from a healthcare professional.

4. **Topical Preparations**: Apply stinging nettle-infused creams, lotions, or ointments to the skin to relieve inflammation, itching, and irritation linked with conditions such as eczema, psoriasis, and insect bites. Ensure products contain high-quality stinging nettle extract for optimal effectiveness.

When harvesting fresh stinging nettle, wear gloves to shield hands from stinging hairs, and handle leaves with care. Use immediately or dry for future use in teas, culinary dishes, or herbal remedies.

Garlic

Garlic, or Allium sativum, with a strong aroma and flavor, is common in cuisines worldwide and revered for its culinary and medicinal properties.

Its anti-inflammatory qualities arises from sulfur compounds like allicin, which inhibit inflammatory enzymes and molecules, thereby reducing inflammation and alleviating symptoms linked to arthritis, cardiovascular disease, and respiratory issues.

To leverage garlic's anti-inflammatory benefits, try:

1. **Raw Garlic**: Crush or chop fresh cloves and allow them to rest briefly to activate beneficial compounds. Incorporate raw garlic into salad dressings, dips, or spreads for both flavor and health advantages.
2. **Cooked Garlic**: Introduce garlic into sauces, soups, stir-fries, and roasted vegetables during cooking. Cooking softens its intensity while preserving therapeutic qualities, enhancing dishes with its versatility.
3. **Garlic Supplements**: Choose garlic extract capsules or tablets for convenient consumption, providing

concentrated garlic compounds supporting daily health and well-being.
4. **Garlic Oil**: Apply garlic-infused oil topically to alleviate inflammation and foster wound healing. Massaging garlic oil onto affected areas offers soothing relief.
5. **Garlic Preparations**: Experiment with homemade remedies like garlic honey, vinegar, and paste, whether for internal consumption or external application, effectively addressing various health concerns, including inflammation and immune support.

Cardamom

Cardamom, or Elettaria cardamomum, is a spice native to the Indian subcontinent and Indonesia, belonging to the ginger family. It boasts a sweet, aromatic flavor with hints of citrus and mint, and is widely used in culinary dishes, beverages, and traditional medicine practices.

Its anti-inflammatory properties are attributed to bioactive compounds like cineole, terpinene, and limonene, which inhibit the production of inflammatory molecules and enzymes, thereby alleviating symptoms associated with arthritis, digestive issues, and respiratory ailments.

To harness cardamom's anti-inflammatory effects, use:

1. **Cardamom Tea**: Brew a soothing tea by steeping crushed cardamom pods or ground seeds in hot water. Enjoy plain or with honey and lemon for added flavor and health benefits.
2. **Culinary Use**: Incorporate cardamom into cooking and baking by adding it to savory dishes, desserts, sauces, and marinades. Its warm and fragrant aroma enhances

both sweet and savory recipes, making it a versatile spice.
3. **Spice Blends**: Create custom spice blends by combining cardamom with other anti-inflammatory spices like turmeric, ginger, and cinnamon. Use these blends to season meats, vegetables, grains, and legumes for flavorful and healthful meals.
4. **Cardamom Infusions**: Infuse cardamom into warm milk or plant-based alternatives for a comforting beverage. Add ground cardamom or crushed pods to milk, heat gently, and sweeten to taste for a cozy and soothing drink.
5. **Cardamom Supplements**: Consider cardamom supplements in capsule or extract form to support overall health and well-being. Consult with a healthcare professional for appropriate dosage and suitability.

Cinnamon

Cinnamon, derived from the inner bark of Cinnamomum trees, is renowned for its warm, sweet flavor and distinctive aroma and is widely used in culinary dishes worldwide. It comes in two main varieties: Ceylon cinnamon and Cassia cinnamon.

Its anti-inflammatory properties stem from bioactive compounds like cinnamaldehyde, cinnamic acid, and cinnamate, which inhibit the production of pro-inflammatory molecules and enzymes, thereby alleviating symptoms associated with arthritis, diabetes, and cardiovascular disease.

To harness cinnamon's anti-inflammatory effects, try:

1. **Cinnamon Tea**: Steep cinnamon sticks or ground powder in hot water for a fragrant tea. Enjoy plain or with honey and lemon juice for added flavor and health benefits.

2. **Culinary Use**: Add cinnamon to oatmeal, smoothies, baked goods, curries, stews, and roasted vegetables to enhance flavor while potentially providing anti-inflammatory benefits.
3. **Spice Blends**: Create homemade spice blends with cinnamon, turmeric, ginger, and cloves. Use these blends to season meats, poultry, fish, vegetables, and legumes for a delicious and healthful twist.
4. **Cinnamon Supplements**: Consider cinnamon supplements in capsule or extract form to support overall health. Consult a healthcare professional for appropriate dosage and suitability.
5. **Topical Applications**: Mix ground cinnamon with honey or coconut oil to create a soothing paste. Apply to inflamed areas of the skin to reduce redness, swelling, and discomfort associated with inflammatory skin conditions.

Chili (Cayenne)

Cayenne pepper, also known as chili, is a hot and spicy variety of Capsicum annuum, recognized for its fiery heat and vibrant red color. Widely used in culinary dishes worldwide, cayenne pepper adds both heat and flavor to various cuisines.

Its anti-inflammatory properties are attributed to capsaicin, the compound responsible for its spicy heat. Capsaicin reduces inflammation by inhibiting certain substances in the body that promote inflammation, potentially aiding in managing conditions such as arthritis and muscle pain.

To harness cayenne's anti-inflammatory effects, try:

1. **Culinary Use**: Add cayenne pepper to soups, stews, sauces, marinades, and stir-fries to infuse heat and flavor into dishes. Start with a small amount and adjust to taste due to its intense spiciness.
2. **Cayenne Tea**: Prepare a soothing tea by adding a pinch of cayenne pepper, lemon juice, and honey to hot water for a warming beverage with potential anti-inflammatory effects.
3. **Topical Application**: Create a homemade paste by mixing ground cayenne pepper with a neutral oil like coconut oil. Apply the paste to areas experiencing inflammation or muscle soreness for relief.
4. **Cayenne Supplements**: Consider cayenne pepper supplements in capsule form for convenient incorporation of anti-inflammatory properties into your daily routine. Follow dosage recommendations and consult a healthcare professional if needed.
5. **Incorporate into Salves and Balms**: Blend cayenne pepper with soothing ingredients like beeswax and shea butter to make homemade salves and balms. These topical preparations can be applied to sore muscles and joints for inflammation and discomfort relief.

HOW TO USE ANTI-INFLAMMATORY PLANTS TOPICALLY

Anti-inflammatory plants may be applied topically to effectively address localized inflammation. Certain plants, such as aloe vera and chamomile, possess soothing properties that calm irritated skin and reduce redness. Applying plant-based remedies such as these directly to the affected area may help alleviate discomfort and promote healing.

Remember to perform a patch test before widespread application to ensure you don't have any adverse reactions. Try a small amount on a small patch of skin and watch out for any adverse effects.

Incorporating topical anti-inflammatory plants into your skincare treatment can offer a natural approach to managing skin inflammation and supporting skin health. The following are some of the most popular topical anti-inflammatory herbal remedies.

Infused Oil With Garlic, Chili, and Ginger

This infused oil with garlic, chili, and ginger adds delicious flavor to your cooking while infusing dishes with potential health benefits. Additionally, the infused oil can be transformed into a soothing topical salve for external use, relieving sore muscles and joints.

Instructions:

1. **Prepare Ingredients**: Peel and crush the garlic cloves. Slice the chili peppers lengthwise, removing seeds for less heat. Slice the ginger root thinly.
2. **Combine Ingredients**: Layer crushed garlic, sliced chili peppers, and ginger in a clean glass jar. Fill the jar with cooking oil, ensuring ingredients are fully submerged.
3. **Infusion Process**: Seal the jar tightly and gently shake to mix. Place the jar in a cool, dark place for 1-2 weeks to infuse flavors. Shake occasionally to redistribute ingredients.

4. **Strain the Oil**: After infusion, strain the oil using a fine mesh sieve or cheesecloth. Press solids to extract infused oil.
5. **Store the Infused Oil**: Transfer the strained oil to clean, sterilized glass bottles with airtight lids. Store in a cool, dry place away from sunlight to maintain freshness.
6. **Optional: Create a Topical Salve**: Combine oil with melted beeswax (4 parts oil to 1 part beeswax). Gently heat mixture in a double boiler until beeswax melts. Pour into clean containers or tins and allow to cool and solidify before use.

Nettle Salves

Nettle salves can be used topically to soothe and nourish the skin, making them ideal for addressing dryness, irritation, and inflammation. Apply the salve to clean, dry skin as needed, gently massaging it into the affected areas.

As with any herbal product, discontinue use if irritation occurs, and consult a healthcare professional if you have any concerns or adverse reactions.

Instructions:

1. **Prepare the Nettle Infusion (if not using dried nettle leaves)**: Combine dried nettle leaves with a carrier oil in a glass jar. Let the mixture infuse in a warm, sunny spot for several weeks, shaking occasionally.
2. **Create the Salve Base**: Melt beeswax and a carrier oil in a double boiler or heat-safe bowl over simmering water. Use a ratio of about 4 parts carrier oil to 1 part beeswax for a firm salve.

3. **Add Nettle Infusion**: Once the beeswax is melted, add the nettle-infused oil to the mixture. Stir well to ensure even distribution throughout the salve base.
4. **Optional: Add Essential Oils**: Incorporate a few drops of chosen essential oils for fragrance and therapeutic benefits. Stir the essential oils into the salve base until well combined.
5. **Pour and Cool**: Carefully pour the warm salve mixture into clean, sterilized containers or tins. Allow the salve to cool and solidify at room temperature before sealing with lids.
6. **Label and Store**: Label containers with the date and contents of the salve. Store nettle salves in a cool, dry place away from direct sunlight to maintain potency and extend shelf life.

Nettle and Devil's Claw Decoction/Compress

Combining stinging nettle and devil's claw in a decoction can create a potent herbal remedy with potential benefits for various health conditions.

Always consult with a healthcare professional before incorporating new herbs into your wellness routine, especially if you have existing health concerns or are taking medications.

Instructions:

1. **Measure Ingredients**: Decide on the desired ratio of stinging nettle to devil's claw based on intended use and potency. Measure the appropriate amount of dried stinging nettle leaves and dried devil's claw root according to the chosen ratio.

2. **Prepare the Herbs**: Place the measured herbs in a clean, dry pot or saucepan.
3. **Add Water**: Pour filtered water into the pot, ensuring the herbs are fully covered with enough water for boiling.
4. **Boil the Decoction**: Put the pot on the stove over medium heat and bring the water to a gentle boil. Reduce heat to low and let the herbs simmer for 20 to 30 minutes to extract beneficial compounds.
5. **Strain the Decoction**: After simmering, remove the pot from heat and let the decoction cool slightly. Strain the liquid through a fine mesh sieve or cheesecloth into a clean container, pressing herbs to extract maximum liquid.
6. **Discard or Reuse the Herbs**: Discard used herbs or compost them. Alternatively, reuse them for another infusion if potency remains.
7. **Store and Use**: Transfer the strained decoction into a clean glass jar or bottle with a tight lid. Store in the refrigerator for several days or freeze in ice cube trays for longer storage. Consume as needed, following recommended dosages for health needs.

HEALING INFLAMMATION YOU CAN'T SEE

Some inflammations are not immediately visible to the naked eye, yet they can still cause discomfort and health issues internally. Incorporating herbal remedies into your cooking can proactively tap into their healing properties and address inflammation from within.

Herbs such as turmeric, ginger, and garlic contain compounds known for their anti-inflammatory effects and can be easily included in various dishes. Integrating these herbs into your meals can support your body's natural healing processes and potentially reduce inflammation systemically.

The following herbal preparations can help boost the body's inflammatory response and promote wellness.

Devil's Claw and Turmeric Tincture

Combining turmeric and devil's claw roots in a tincture can create a potent herbal remedy with potential anti-inflammatory properties. Always consult with a healthcare practitioner before incorporating new herbs or supplements into your wellness routine, especially if you have underlying health conditions or are taking medications.

Instructions:

1. **Prepare the Roots**: Clean fresh turmeric root thoroughly to remove dirt or debris. Peel and chop turmeric root into small pieces. Measure out dried devil's claw root according to desired ratio for the tincture.
2. **Combine Herbs and Alcohol**: Place chopped turmeric and dried devil's claw root in the glass jar. Pour enough high-proof alcohol over the herbs to cover completely, with at least an inch of alcohol above them.
3. **Seal and Shake**: Tighten the jar lid securely and shake vigorously to mix the herbs and alcohol.
4. **Infusion Period**: Store the sealed jar in a cool, dark place like a kitchen cabinet or pantry. Let the herbs steep in alcohol for 4 to 6 weeks, shaking gently every few days to agitate the mixture and promote extraction of herbal compounds.
5. **Strain the Tincture**: After the infusion period, strain the tincture using cheesecloth or a fine mesh sieve to separate

liquid from solid herbs. Squeeze the herbs to extract as much liquid as possible.
6. **Bottle and Store**: Transfer the strained tincture into clean, sterilized glass bottles or jars with tight-fitting lids. Label each bottle with the preparation date and contents. Store the tincture in a cool, dark place away from direct sunlight to maintain potency.

Cinnamon Tea

Cinnamon tea is not only delicious but also offers potential health benefits, including anti-inflammatory and antioxidant properties. Incorporate it into your daily routine for a soothing and flavorful beverage.

Instructions:

1. **Prepare Cinnamon**: Break cinnamon sticks into smaller pieces to increase surface area and flavor exposure. Measure the desired amount of ground cinnamon based on taste preferences.
2. **Boil Water**: Bring filtered water to a boil in a pot or kettle.
3. **Add Cinnamon**: Once the water boils, add cinnamon sticks or ground cinnamon to the pot. Use about 1 to 2 cinnamon sticks or 1 to 2 teaspoons of ground cinnamon per 8 ounces of water.
4. **Steep Cinnamon**: Turn off the heat and cover pot. Let the cinnamon steep in hot water for 10 to 15 minutes, adjusting steeping time for preferred flavor intensity.
5. **Strain and Serve**: After steeping, strain the cinnamon tea to remove any particles or debris. Pour the tea into cups or mugs.

6. **Optional Flavorings**: Enhance flavor with honey, lemon juice, or other desired flavorings. Stir well to blend flavors.

GENERAL IMMUNE SYSTEM BOOSTERS

Some medicinal plants are immune system boosters, aiding your quest for overall wellness. Incorporating these plants into your routine can support your body's natural defenses against illness and infection.

You can proactively support your health and vitality by harnessing the power of immune-boosting plants. The following are examples of the best immune system-boosting plants.

Echinacea

Echinacea, or purple coneflower, native to North America, is part of the Asteraceae family, known for its purple petals and cone-shaped center. It boosts the immune system with active compounds like alkamides, polysaccharides, and flavonoids, aiding in fighting infections.

Echinacea is available in capsules, tablets, or tinctures. Echinacea tea brewed from dried roots or leaves can also enhance immune health when consumed regularly during periods of susceptibility to illness.

Elder

Elder, scientifically known as Sambucus nigra, hails from Europe, North America, and parts of Asia, featuring clusters of small, white, or cream-colored flowers and dark-purple berries. Renowned for their immune-boosting properties, elderberries are rich in antioxidants, especially flavonoids like anthocyanins, along with vitamins A, B, and C, and minerals such as potassium and iron, bolstering immune function and combating oxidative stress.

To use elder's benefits, options include elderberry syrup or tea from dried berries for daily consumption, alongside elderberry supplements, available in capsule or liquid form, particularly useful during colder seasons. Integrating elderberries into your diet and supplements promotes immune resilience and overall well-being.

Goldenseal

Goldenseal, scientifically named Hydrastis canadensis, is a perennial herb native to the eastern United States and Canada, recognized by its vibrant yellow rhizomes and knotted roots. It has been historically used by Native American tribes for its medicinal attributes.

This herb comes with immune-boosting qualities because of berberine, an alkaloid compound that boasts antimicrobial and anti-inflammatory properties, aiding the body's immune response against harmful pathogens like bacteria, viruses, and fungi. Hence, goldenseal is widely favored for enhancing overall immune health.

Goldenseal is available in dietary supplements, including capsules, tablets, or liquid extracts. Additionally, goldenseal tea, crafted from dried goldenseal root or rhizome, provides another means to access its medicinal advantages. However, it's essential to use goldenseal responsibly and seek advice from a healthcare professional before integration, as excessive or prolonged usage may yield adverse effects.

Reishi Mushrooms

Reishi mushrooms, or Ganoderma lucidum, are fungi from the Polyporaceae family, native to Asian regions like China, Japan, and Korea. Recognized by their reddish-brown caps and woody texture, they've long been esteemed in traditional Chinese medicine for their medicinal qualities.

Reishi mushrooms boast immune-boosting properties because of polysaccharides, triterpenes, and other bioactive compounds. These regulate the immune system and boosts its defense against infections and diseases. Furthermore, reishi mushrooms offer antioxidant benefits, shielding cells from free radicals and oxidative stress.

These mushrooms are available in diverse forms such as dietary supplements, including capsules, tablets, or powdered extracts. Reishi mushroom tea, crafted from dried slices or powder, provides another avenue to tap into their benefits. Additionally, integrating reishi mushrooms into savory dishes like soups and stews enhances both flavor and nutritional content. Regular consumption can contribute to overall immune health and well-being.

CONCLUSION

A healthy immune system helps the body recognize and fight off pathogens, such as bacteria and viruses, reducing infections. A strong immune system maintains overall health. These herbal immune boosters can boost immune system functions, fight infections, and preserve health.

Do you know how much more you can achieve in a day with more energy? The next chapter is about Energizing Adaptogens, E in the HERBS framework. Adaptogens help you handle stress and improve the cardiovascular system, giving you more energy and vitality. So let's meet in Chapter 5!

The Herbal Route to Peace of Mind

"A man may esteem himself happy when that which is his food is also his medicine."

— HENRY DAVID THOREAU

Remember Akosua, who I told you about in the introduction? Her knowledge and understanding of herbs allowed her to take care of her own health during pregnancy, something she was able to do without any extra research. Imagine the peace of mind in that. That's the peace of mind you're cultivating for yourself as you learn more about the power of herbal remedies and the secrets held by the natural world.

It may still feel a little overwhelming at this point – after all, you're taking in a lot of new information. But rest assured that, over time, your confidence will grow, and herbal healing will become second nature to you. That's hugely empowering. It doesn't mean that you'll never have any need for modern medicine again, but it does mean that you'll have the skills and knowledge you need to battle common ailments and take proactive steps to keep your health in check before any hint of an illness begins to make itself known.

For Akosua, this was knowledge that was part of her culture. It was wisdom that she grew up with, and something she always had at her fingertips. This is something we could have too, and my mission in writing this book was to make these skills accessible to more people... and this is where I'd like to ask for your help.

A book is only useful when it reaches the hands of the people who are looking for the information it contains, and to make that happen, it must have reviews. That's something you can help with by taking just a few minutes to write your own.

By leaving a review of this book on Amazon, you'll show new readers exactly where they can find all the wisdom about herbal remedies that they're looking for – and that's a sure route to peace of mind when it comes to their health.

Reviews are what help to circulate books, so while it may not seem like much to you, the few minutes you spend doing this will make a huge difference.

Thank you so much for your support: It's as powerful as the herbs themselves.

E: ENERGIZING ADAPTOGENS

Ever felt weighed down by stress and fatigue, struggling to stay active and energized? Exercise is vital for a healthy heart, but life often gets in the way.

That's where adaptogens come in. These help your body handle stress and keep balance. But here's the key: This isn't just about relieving stress and anxiety, though adaptogens can help with those too. Our focus is on your cardiovascular health.

Michael Phelps once said, "The problem with heart disease is that the first symptom is often fatal." Your heart works tirelessly, silently, day and night. It deserves attention. While exercise is crucial, daily stress and low energy levels can make it hard to keep up a healthy lifestyle.

Adaptogens do more than relieve stress. They improve blood circulation, ensuring your organs get oxygen. They also regulate blood pressure, reducing strain on your heart.

As you learn about adaptogens and their impact on cardiovascular health, remember: It's not just about finding remedies. It's about embracing a holistic approach to caring for your heart and body. This can foster lasting vitality and resilience, empowering you to live your best life.

WHAT TO EXPECT WHEN MORE OXYGEN FLOWS IN YOUR BLOOD

Improving blood flow and oxygenation brings remarkable benefits. Enhanced circulation speeds up healing and recovery, helping you bounce back from an injury or illness. Nutrients reach where they're needed swiftly, promoting quicker and stronger recuperation.

Maintaining good blood flow ensures vitality and wellness. Like nourishing a plant, sufficient oxygen and nutrients invigorate your body, leaving you energized and prepared for challenges.

Smooth blood flow and optimal oxygen levels benefit your entire body. Muscles perform better, the mind feels sharper, and skin appears healthier. It's like giving your body a tune-up for seamless functioning.

Remember, enhancing blood flow and oxygenation isn't solely for recovery; it's about feeling your best every day, fostering strength and resilience.

ADAPTOGENS TO HELP YOU RELAX

Adaptogens help restore balance within your body and mind, allowing you to navigate through life's turbulence with greater ease. As you incorporate adaptogens into your routine, you'll notice a gradual but profound shift in your ability to unwind and find tranquility amid the hustle and bustle of daily life.

These work harmoniously with your body, fostering a sense of calm and serenity that allows you to embrace moments of peace amid the chaos. Here are the best herbal adaptogens.

Chamomile

Chamomile, Matricaria chamomilla or Chamaemelum nobile, is a daisy-like herb hailing from the Asteraceae family. Native to Europe, Western Asia, and North Africa, its cultivation has spread worldwide. Chamomile boasts delicate white petals with a yellow center, emitting a delightful, apple-like scent.

Famed for its relaxing properties, chamomile harbors compounds like apigenin, which engage brain receptors to induce relaxation and diminish stress and anxiety. Often sought to soothe nerves, enhance sleep quality, and relieve tension, chamomile is a go-to remedy for calmness.

To tap into chamomile's tranquil effects, various avenues are available. Chamomile tea, a popular choice, involves steeping dried chamomile flowers in hot water, ideal for evening relaxation and improved sleep. Alternatively, chamomile essential oil, when diluted, can be topically applied or diffused in aromatherapy to foster a serene ambiance. Introducing chamomile into daily routines can aid in stress relief and overall well-being.

Lavender

Lavender, or Lavandula angustifolia, is a fragrant plant from the Lamiaceae family, native to the Mediterranean but grown worldwide for its scent and healing properties. Its slender flowers and silvery-green leaves define its appearance.

It contains compounds like linalool and linalyl acetate, which soothe the nervous system, reducing stress, anxiety, and tension for enhanced relaxation and well-being.

To enjoy lavender's tranquility, various options are available. Lavender essential oil is versatile, perfect for diffusers, massage oils, or bathwater, offering a calming experience. Lavender tea, crafted from dried flowers, enhances relaxation and sleep quality. Lavender sachets, placed under pillows or in drawers, release a soothing aroma, promoting tranquility in the environment. Adding lavender into daily routines aids stress relief and promotes serenity.

Lemon Balm

Lemon balm, or Melissa officinalis, is a lemon-scented herb from the mint family, Lamiaceae. Originally from Europe, North Africa, and West Asia, it's now grown worldwide for its culinary and medicinal benefits, featuring bright-green leaves and small white flowers.

Valued for its calming properties, lemon balm contains compounds like rosmarinic acid and flavonoids, gently soothing the nervous system. It's commonly used to ease anxiety, induce relaxation, and uplift mood, popular for stress-relieving herbal remedies.

To enjoy lemon balm's calming effects, it can be consumed as tea, made by steeping dried or fresh leaves in hot water. This tea promotes calmness and releases tension throughout the day. Additionally, lemon balm essential oil, when diluted, can be applied to pulse points or diffused in aromatherapy to create a serene environment. Regular use of lemon balm supports overall relaxation and well-being.

Holy Basil

Holy basil, also known as Ocimum sanctum or Ocimum tenuiflorum, is a revered herb cultivated in India and Southeast Asia. It's cherished for both its religious significance and medicinal benefits. Holy basil, belonging to the Lamiaceae family, is known for its aromatic leaves with a peppery flavor, widely used in cooking and herbal remedies.

Recognized for its calming effects, holy basil contains compounds like eugenol and caryophyllene that soothe the nervous system. It's commonly utilized to alleviate stress, anxiety, and fatigue, fostering relaxation and mental clarity.

To experience the relaxing properties of holy basil, it can be consumed as tea, prepared by steeping fresh or dried leaves in hot water. This tea offers relaxation and well-being throughout the day. Additionally, holy basil essential oil, when diluted, can be used in aromatherapy diffusers or applied to pulse points for its calming scent. Adding holy basil to your daily routine can ease stress and cultivate a sense of tranquility and balance.

Catnip

Catnip, or Nepeta cataria, belongs to the mint family and is native to Europe and Asia. It's a perennial herb with heart-shaped leaves and small flowers in white or purple. Catnip emits a distinct aroma that attracts cats, but it also offers medicinal benefits recognized for centuries.

This herb also acts as a mild sedative for humans. It contains nepetalactone, a compound that naturally relaxes. This helps reduce anxiety, induce relaxation, and promote sleepiness in some people.

To experience catnip's relaxing effects, you can make catnip tea by steeping dried leaves in hot water. Drinking this tea before bedtime can enhance relaxation and sleep quality. Catnip essential oil, when diluted, can be used in aromatherapy diffusers or applied to pulse points for its calming properties. Adding catnip to your relaxation routine can ease stress and foster a sense of tranquility.

Valerian

Valerian, scientifically named Valeriana officinalis, is a perennial plant native to Europe and parts of Asia, recognized by its tall stems, compound leaves, and clusters of small white or pink flowers. Valerian root is the part most commonly used for its medicinal benefits.

Valerian is celebrated for its calming properties, containing compounds like valerenic acid and valeranone that interact with brain neurotransmitters to induce relaxation and ease anxiety. It's often used to ease insomnia, anxiety, and restlessness, making it a popular remedy for better sleep and overall relaxation.

To experience valerian's calming effects, you can make valerian root tea by steeping dried root in hot water. Drinking this tea before bedtime can promote relaxation and improve sleep. Valerian supplements, available in capsules or tinctures, can also be used as directed to help reduce anxiety and foster calmness. Adding valerian to your relaxation routine can bolster mental and emotional well-being.

HOW TO GIVE YOUR HEART AN ENERGY BOOST

Give your heart a boost with adaptogenic plants and herbs. These plants support cardiovascular health by reducing stress, improving circulation, and enhancing overall heart function. You can enjoy them through teas, tinctures, or supplements to give your heart the natural energy it needs to thrive.

Rosemary

Rosemary, scientifically named Rosmarinus officinalis, is a fragrant herb from the mint family, Lamiaceae, native to the Mediterranean but grown globally for its culinary and medicinal uses. Recognizable by its needle-like leaves and small blue flowers, rosemary is prized for its robust flavor and aromatic scent.

Rosemary boasts heart-healthy properties due to compounds like rosmarinic acid and carnosic acid, which possess antioxidant and anti-inflammatory effects. These properties combat oxidative stress and inflammation, benefiting cardiovascular health. Rosemary also aids circulation and supports healthy blood pressure levels.

To enjoy rosemary's cardiovascular benefits, include it in your diet by adding fresh or dried leaves to dishes like roasted vegetables, meats, and soups. You can also brew rosemary tea by steeping the leaves in hot water for a soothing drink. Rosemary essential oil, when diluted, can be used in aromatherapy or applied topically to promote relaxation and reduce stress, further supporting heart health. Making rosemary a part of your daily routine can enhance your heart health and overall well-being.

Hawthorn

Hawthorn, scientifically known as Crataegus laevigata or monogyna, is a shrub or small tree found in Europe, North America, and Asia, recognized by its white or pink flowers and small red berries. With a rich history in traditional medicine, hawthorn is revered for its heart health benefits.

Hawthorn positively impacts cardiovascular health due to its potent antioxidants and flavonoids. These compounds strengthen blood vessels, enhance circulation, and support overall heart function. Hawthorn promotes healthy blood pressure and cholesterol levels while improving the heart's pumping efficiency, making it vital for heart health maintenance.

To enjoy hawthorn's benefits, prepare hawthorn tea by steeping dried berries or leaves in hot water. Regular consumption of hawthorn tea can support heart health. Alternatively, hawthorn supplements, available in capsules, extracts, or tinctures, can complement a heart-healthy lifestyle when taken as directed by a healthcare professional. Embracing hawthorn in your daily routine can foster a healthier heart and better cardiovascular function.

Parsley

Parsley, scientifically named Petroselinum crispum, is a renowned culinary herb originating from the Mediterranean and now grown globally. It belongs to the Apiaceae family, recognizable by its lush green, finely serrated leaves, and petite white flowers. Praised for its refreshing taste and scent, parsley is a staple in many dishes worldwide.

Parsley boasts heart-healthy attributes owing to its rich nutrient profile, including vitamins C, K, and folate, alongside flavonoids and antioxidants like luteolin and apigenin. These components aid in maintaining blood vessel integrity, curbing inflammation, and neutralizing free radicals that could harm heart tissues. Regular parsley consumption may contribute to lowering cholesterol, managing blood pressure, and enhancing overall heart function.

To leverage parsley's cardiovascular benefits, integrate fresh parsley leaves into daily meals, from salads and soups to sauces and smoothies. You can also brew herbal teas by steeping fresh or dried parsley leaves in hot water. Alternatively, parsley supplements, available in capsule or extract forms, offer a convenient method to augment heart-healthy nutrients in your diet. Embracing parsley as part of a balanced lifestyle can promote heart health and overall vitality.

Black Pepper

Black pepper, scientifically named Piper nigrum, is a vine renowned for its dried fruit, widely used as a spice globally. Originating from South India, it belongs to the Piperaceae family and is esteemed for its bold taste and aroma, enhancing a broad spectrum of dishes.

In black pepper lies piperine, a bioactive compound bestowing its distinctive flavor and manifold health benefits. Piperine exhibits potential in promoting cardiovascular wellness by improving blood circulation, mitigating inflammation, and reducing cholesterol levels. Moreover, black pepper boasts antioxidants that shield heart cells from oxidative stress, bolstering heart health.

To harness black pepper's cardiovascular benefits, integrate it into daily cooking. Sprinkle freshly ground black pepper onto salads, soups, stews, marinades, and other savory creations to elevate taste and nurture heart health. Alternatively, savor black pepper tea by infusing crushed peppercorns in hot water for a calming, invigorating beverage. Embracing black pepper in culinary ventures emerges as a seamless and delightful approach to boost cardiovascular function and overall vitality.

TAKING CARE OF YOUR BLOOD PRESSURE

Adaptogenic herbs help you manage your blood pressure and promote cardiovascular health. Adaptogens help the body adapt to stressors and maintain balance. Incorporating these herbs into your daily routine supports your body's natural ability to regulate blood pressure levels and promote overall cardiovascular health.

Basil

Basil, scientifically termed Ocimum basilicum, is a fragrant herb from the Lamiaceae family. Originating from tropical areas in Asia and Africa, basil is now cultivated globally for its culinary and medicinal values. Its distinct aroma and taste make basil a kitchen essential, celebrated for its adaptability and health perks.

In basil are eugenol, linalool, and flavonoids, compounds explored for their potential in supporting heart health and blood pressure regulation. These elements help in relaxing blood vessels, enhancing blood circulation, and mitigating hypertension, fostering overall cardiovascular well-being. Regular consumption of fresh or dried basil can complement a wholesome diet and lifestyle to maintain optimal blood pressure levels.

To leverage basil's cardiovascular advantages, add it to daily meals. Sprinkle fresh basil leaves onto salads, sandwiches, pasta, and soups. Enjoy basil-infused beverages like herbal teas or infused water for a refreshing twist and heart-healthy boost. Consider cultivating basil in a pot or garden for convenient access to fresh leaves. By embracing basil in your culinary ventures, you can proactively manage blood pressure and nurture cardiovascular health.

Thyme

Thyme, scientifically named Thymus vulgaris, is a fragrant herb originating from the Mediterranean and southern Europe. Belonging to the Lamiaceae family, thyme boasts small, aromatic leaves and delicate flowers, cherished for its unique flavor and potential health perks.

Within thyme are bioactive compounds like rosmarinic acid, flavonoids, and volatile oils, studied for their role in supporting heart health and regulating blood pressure. These components may aid in widening blood vessels, enhancing circulation, and reducing hypertension, nurturing overall cardiovascular well-being. Regular inclusion of fresh or dried thyme in your diet can complement a healthy lifestyle, maintaining optimal blood pressure levels.

To tap into thyme's cardiovascular advantages, infuse it into your daily meals. Sprinkle fresh or dried thyme leaves onto roasted meats, vegetables, soups, and sauces for enhanced taste and heart support. Thyme can also be brewed into herbal teas or infused into vinegar for added health benefits. Cultivate thyme in pots or gardens for easy access to fresh leaves year-round. By embracing thyme in your culinary endeavors, you actively promote blood pressure management and bolster overall cardiovascular health.

Celery Seeds

Celery seeds, extracted from the celery plant (Apium graveolens), offer a distinct flavor and potential health advantages. While celery stalks are common in cooking and salads, celery seeds are prized for their slightly bitter taste and health perks, used as both a spice and herbal remedy in various cuisines and traditional medicines.

Rich in compounds like phthalides, coumarins, and flavonoids, celery seeds bolster cardiovascular health and manage blood pressure. These elements relax blood vessels, enhance circulation, and regulate blood pressure, fostering overall heart well-being. Regular incorporation of celery seeds, whether whole or ground, complements a wholesome diet and lifestyle aimed at sustaining balanced blood pressure levels.

To harness the cardiovascular advantages of celery seeds, infuse them into your dishes and diets. Use them as seasoning in savory dishes, soups, stews, and salads to enrich flavor and texture. Alternatively, brew celery seed tea by steeping crushed seeds in hot water for a calming and aromatic drink. For extra taste and nutrition, grind celery seeds and sprinkle them over roasted veggies or grilled meats. By integrating celery seeds into your meals, you improve your cardiovascular system and promote heart health overall.

Ginger

Ginger, or Zingiber officinale, hails from Southeast Asia, renowned for its aromatic rhizome and cherished both as a spice and an herbal remedy. Its robust, slightly spicy flavor enriches a variety of dishes and beverages, reflecting its rich history in traditional medicine and culinary traditions globally.

In terms of cardiovascular health, ginger boasts bioactive compounds like gingerol, shogaol, and paradol, explored for their potential to bolster heart health and regulate blood pressure. These compounds aid in dilating blood vessels, enhancing circulation, and managing blood pressure levels, contributing to overall cardiovascular wellness. Regular incorporation of ginger, whether fresh, dried, or powdered, complements a balanced diet, fostering healthy blood pressure levels and heart function.

To benefit from ginger's cardiovascular effects, add it into your daily diet and wellness practices. Enhance teas, soups, stir-fries, smoothies, and baked goods with fresh ginger slices or grated ginger for a zesty kick. Opt for ginger tea by steeping fresh slices in hot water or relish ginger-infused water for a revitalizing drink. Elevate marinades, dressings, and sauces with ginger to enrich flavor and nutritional value. By embracing ginger in your culinary ventures, you fortify your cardiovascular system and nurture overall heart health.

SIMPLE RECIPES FOR HEART HEALTH AND ENERGY

The following are simple recipes using adaptogenic herbs to boost heart health and promote energy levels.

Ginger and Hawthorn Tincture Syrup

A ginger and hawthorn tincture syrup combines the warming properties of ginger with the cardiovascular support of hawthorn berries. This remedy is easy to make and offers both flavor and health benefits.

Instructions:

1. **Prepare Ingredients**: Gather 2-3 pieces of 1-inch ginger and hawthorn berries.
2. **Combine With Alcohol**: Place the ginger pieces and hawthorn berries in a jar and cover them with alcohol, such as vodka or brandy.
3. **Steep**: Seal the jar and let the mixture steep for several weeks in a cool, dark place to allow the flavors and properties to infuse.
4. **Strain**: After steeping, strain the liquid to remove the ginger pieces and hawthorn berries.
5. **Create Syrup**: Mix the strained liquid with honey or sugar to create a syrup, adjusting the sweetness to taste.
6. **Store**: Pour the ginger and hawthorn syrup into a clean bottle or jar and store it in the refrigerator for future use.

Remember not to discard the hawthorn berries after making the tincture! Instead, consider repurposing them into salsa for a delicious and nutritious treat. However, be cautious and remove as many seeds as possible from the hawthorn berries, as they contain cyanide, similar to apple pips. By being mindful of seed removal, you can enjoy the benefits of hawthorn berries while ensuring safety in your culinary creations.

Catnip and Lemon Balm Tea

Catnip and lemon balm tea is a soothing herbal infusion known for its calming properties and refreshing flavor. This tea blend combines the mild, minty taste of catnip with the citrusy aroma of lemon balm, creating a delightful beverage ideal for relaxation and enjoyment.

Instructions:

1. **Gather Ingredients**: Obtain dried catnip leaves and dried lemon balm leaves.
2. **Combine Herbs**: Mix equal parts of dried catnip and lemon balm leaves in a tea infuser or teapot.
3. **Boil Water**: Heat water in a kettle until it reaches a rolling boil.
4. **Infuse Tea**: Place the tea infuser or herbs directly into a teapot and pour the boiling water over them.
5. **Steep**: Allow the herbs to steep in the hot water for 5-7 minutes to extract their flavors and beneficial properties.
6. **Strain and Serve**: After steeping, remove the tea infuser or strain the tea to remove the herbs. Pour the infused tea into cups and serve hot.
7. **Optional Additions**: Sweeten the tea with honey or add a splash of lemon juice for extra flavor, if desired.
8. **Enjoy**: Savor the calming and refreshing qualities of catnip and lemon balm tea as you relax and unwind.

This simple herbal tea is perfect for enjoying throughout the day or as a bedtime beverage to promote relaxation and tranquility.

Thyme and Rosemary Decoction

A thyme and rosemary decoction is a potent herbal infusion known for its aromatic fragrance and therapeutic properties. This herbal blend combines the earthy tones of thyme with the pine-like essence of rosemary, offering a revitalizing and refreshing concoction.

Instructions:

1. **Prepare Ingredients**: Gather fresh or dried thyme sprigs and rosemary sprigs.
2. **Boil Water**: Fill a pot with water and bring it to a boil over medium heat.
3. **Add Herbs**: Add the thyme and rosemary sprigs to the pot once the water reaches a rolling boil.
4. **Simmer**: Reduce the heat to low and allow the herbs to simmer gently in the water for 15-20 minutes.
5. **Strain**: After simmering, remove the pot from the heat and strain the liquid to separate the decoction from the herbs.
6. **Usage Options**:

- **Drink**: Enjoy the decoction as a warm herbal tea to invigorate the senses and promote overall well-being.
- **Bath Additive**: Add the decoction to your bathwater for a soothing and aromatic soak, ideal for relaxation and muscle relief.
- **Foot Bath**: Create a foot bath by adding the decoction to warm water, perfect for soothing tired and achy feet after a long day.

- **Hair Rinse**: Use the decoction as a hair rinse to stimulate blood flow to the scalp, promoting healthy hair growth and scalp health.

Incorporate this versatile thyme and rosemary decoction into your daily routine to experience its rejuvenating benefits for the body, mind, and spirit.

Valerian Root and Celery Seed Tincture

The valerian root and celery seed tincture is a potent herbal extract known for its calming and soothing properties. This tincture offers a natural solution for relaxation and wellness.

Instructions:

1. **Gather Ingredients**: Obtain dried valerian root and celery seeds from a reputable source.
2. **Prepare Jar**: Choose a clean glass jar with a tight-fitting lid for the tincture.
3. **Combine Herbs**: Fill the jar halfway with dried valerian root and celery seeds, ensuring an equal ratio of both herbs.
4. **Add Alcohol**: Pour enough high-proof alcohol (such as vodka or grain alcohol) to completely cover the herbs in the jar.
5. **Seal and Shake**: Seal the jar tightly with the lid and shake it vigorously to thoroughly mix the herbs with the alcohol.
6. **Label and Store**: Label the jar with the date and contents, then store it in a cool, dark place away from direct sunlight.

7. **Infuse**: Allow the herbs to infuse in the alcohol for at least 4-6 weeks, shaking the jar gently every few days to agitate the mixture.
8. **Strain and Bottle**: After infusion, strain the tincture through a fine mesh sieve or cheesecloth to remove the herbal residue.
9. **Bottle and Store**: Transfer the strained tincture into amber glass dropper bottles for convenient use. Store the bottles in a cool, dark place for long-term storage.

Enjoy the calming and balancing effects of the valerian root and celery seed tincture by adding a few drops to water, juice, or herbal tea as needed for relaxation and stress relief.

Holy Basil, Turmeric, and Ginger Tea

The holy basil, turmeric, and ginger tea blend combines the aromatic notes of holy basil with the warming spice of ginger and the earthy undertones of turmeric. This refreshing herbal infusion offers a delightful balance of flavors and myriad health benefits, making it a soothing and comforting beverage.

Instructions:

1. **Prepare Ingredients**: Gather fresh or dried holy basil leaves, turmeric root, and ginger root.
2. **Slice Ingredients**: If using fresh ingredients, thinly slice the turmeric and ginger roots for better infusion.
3. **Boil Water**: Bring a pot of water to a boil over medium heat on the stove.
4. **Add Ingredients**: Once the water reaches a rolling boil, add the holy basil leaves, sliced turmeric, and ginger to the pot.

5. **Simmer**: Reduce the heat to low and allow the herbs and spices to simmer gently in the water for 10-15 minutes.
6. **Steep**: After simmering, remove the pot from the heat and let the tea steep for 5-10 minutes to fully extract the flavors and nutrients.
7. **Strain and Serve**: Use a fine mesh sieve or tea strainer to strain the tea into cups or mugs, discarding the spent herbs and spices.
8. **Optional Additions**: Sweeten the tea with honey or a splash of lemon juice, and garnish with fresh holy basil leaves or a slice of lemon for extra flavor.
9. **Enjoy**: Sip and savor the warm and comforting holy basil, turmeric, and ginger tea, embracing its delightful flavors and nourishing qualities with each sip.

Experience this revitalizing tea's harmonious blend of holy basil, turmeric, and ginger, perfect for promoting overall wellness and vitality.

Homemade Dried Mixed Herbs

Homemade dried mixed herbs are a versatile culinary blend that adds depth and flavor to various dishes. This fragrant combination typically includes basil, parsley, rosemary, and thyme, offering a harmonious balance of aromas and tastes that enhance savory recipes.

Instructions:

1. **Gather Fresh Herbs**: Obtain fresh basil, parsley, rosemary, and thyme from your garden or local market.
2. **Preheat Oven**: Preheat your oven to its lowest setting, typically around 200°F (93°C).

3. **Prepare Herbs**: Rinse the fresh herbs under cold water and gently pat them dry with paper towels to remove excess moisture.
4. **Remove Stems and Chop**: Strip the leaves from the stems and discard the stems. Chop the herbs finely using a sharp knife.
5. **Spread on Baking Sheet**: Spread the chopped herbs evenly on a baking sheet lined with parchment paper, ensuring they are in a single layer and not overlapping.
6. **Dry in Oven**: Place the baking sheet in the oven and allow the herbs to dry slowly for 1-2 hours or until completely dry and brittle.
7. **Check for Dryness**: After the initial drying period, check the herbs for dryness by crumbling a small amount between your fingers. They should be crisp and crush easily.
8. **Cool and Store**: Remove the baking sheet from the oven and let the dried herbs cool completely at room temperature.
9. **Store in Airtight Container**: Once cooled, transfer the dried mixed herbs to an airtight container or glass jar with a tight-fitting lid.
10. **Label and Date**: Label the container with the name of the herbs and the date of preparation for easy identification.
11. **Store in Cool, Dark Place**: Store the homemade dried mixed herbs in a cool, dark place away from direct sunlight to preserve their flavor and aroma.
12. **Use in Recipes**: Enjoy using your homemade dried mixed herbs to season soups, stews, sauces, marinades, and other culinary creations, adding flavor to your favorite dishes.

With this simple homemade dried mixed herbs recipe, you can elevate the taste of your meals and enjoy the convenience of having flavorful herbs on hand whenever you need them.

Valerian Root and Lavender Salve

Valerian root and lavender salve is a soothing herbal remedy that promotes relaxation and eases tension before bedtime. Blending the calming properties of valerian root and lavender, this salve offers a gentle way to unwind and prepare for a restful night's sleep.

Instructions:

1. **Infuse Oil**: Begin by infusing a carrier oil, such as olive or coconut oil, with dried valerian root and lavender flowers. To do this, fill a clean glass jar with the herbs and cover them with the carrier oil. Seal the jar and let it sit in a warm, sunny spot for 2-4 weeks, shaking it gently every few days to encourage infusion.
2. **Strain the Oil**: After the infusion period, strain the oil through a fine mesh sieve or cheesecloth to remove the herbs, ensuring you extract all the infused oil.
3. **Create Salve Base**: In a heat-safe container, combine the infused oil with beeswax pellets or grated beeswax, using approximately 4 parts oil to 1 part beeswax. Adjust the ratio based on desired consistency, adding more beeswax for a firmer salve.
4. **Melt and Blend**: Create a double boiler setup by placing the container with the oil and beeswax over a pot of simmering water. Heat gently until the beeswax melts completely, stirring occasionally to blend the ingredients.

5. **Add Essential Oils (Optional)**: For added fragrance and therapeutic benefits, consider adding a few drops of lavender essential oil to enhance the aroma and relaxation properties of the salve. Stir well to incorporate.
6. **Pour into Containers**: Once fully blended, carefully pour the liquid salve into clean, sterilized jars or tins, filling them to the desired level.
7. **Cool and Solidify**: Allow the salve to cool and solidify at room temperature, which may take several hours. Avoid disturbing the containers during this time to prevent uneven texture.
8. **Usage**: To use the valerian root and lavender salve, simply scoop a small amount onto your fingertips and gently massage your temples and inner wrists before bedtime. Allow the salve's soothing aroma and calming properties to promote relaxation and prepare your mind and body for sleep.

CONCLUSION

With a relaxed body and mind, it's time to move on to lung health and the respiratory system. And, although many of the herbs we have seen so far can help support the respiratory system, there are more to come in Chapter 6. It's time to learn Respiratory Soothers, R in the HERBS framework. Let's go!

R: RESPIRATORY SOOTHERS

Welcome to a chapter where we learn about herbal remedies for your respiratory health! Let's explore how medicinal herbs can give your lungs a helping hand when they're feeling under pressure.

Think about it: Respiratory problems are all around us. Our respiratory systems face various challenges, from annoying allergies to stubborn congestion and persistent coughs. And it's not just the occasional cold or flu that can cause trouble. Chronic lung conditions such as asthma and chronic obstructive pulmonary disease (COPD) affect millions of people, making each breath a bit more challenging.

But fear not! Nature has provided us with a treasure trove of herbs that can relieve and support our respiratory systems. Whether you're dealing with a pesky cold or managing a more severe lung condition, herbs can help ease the pressure and make breathing a little easier.

So, let's dive in and discover which herbs can be your allies in the battle for better respiratory health!

THE DUAL EFFECTS OF HERBAL REMEDIES ON THE LUNGS

Inflammation in the lungs acts as a warning sign of underlying issues. While it's the body's natural response to irritation or infection, chronic inflammation can lead to serious respiratory conditions like asthma and COPD.

Plants with anti-inflammatory properties can help soothe inflammation, reducing swelling and discomfort. By addressing the root cause, these plants offer relief and support for better respiratory health.

Additionally, herbal teas used for steam therapy provide multiple benefits to the respiratory system. Inhaling warm, herb-infused steam helps loosen stubborn mucus in the nasal passages, throat, and lungs, easing breathing and clearing congestion. The soothing warmth also relaxes airways, reducing inflammation and enhancing overall respiratory comfort.

Next time you're congested or battling a cough, consider enjoying a steamy herbal tea session for much-needed respiratory relief.

Stinging Nettle

Stinging nettle, despite its initial sting, offers remarkable properties for managing allergies. When processed correctly, it becomes a potent herbal remedy for alleviating allergy symptoms and promoting well-being.

This herb is known for its stinging hairs. Harvest fresh nettle leaves and infuse them with high-proof alcohol for 4-6 weeks to create a tincture. Strain the liquid, bottle it, and take 1-2 dropperfuls diluted in water or juice up to three times daily during allergy season. Always consult a healthcare professional before use.

By carefully preparing the tincture, you can harness the allergy management properties of stinging nettle to support your overall well-being.

Peppermint

Peppermint, known for its refreshing scent and soothing qualities, offers effective relief for allergies. Brew peppermint tea or inhale steam with peppermint oil to clear nasal passages and ease respiratory discomfort.

Massage diluted peppermint oil onto your chest and temples for headache relief, or use a portable inhaler for quick relief on the go. Incorporate fresh peppermint into your meals cautiously, as it may cause adverse reactions in some individuals. Perform a patch test before using peppermint oil and consult a healthcare professional if you have concerns.

By adding peppermint into your daily routine, you can naturally alleviate seasonal discomfort and promote overall well-being with its powerful allergy-relief properties.

Chamomile

Chamomile, known for its calming scent and anti-inflammatory properties, is a natural remedy for allergy relief. Brew chamomile tea to ease symptoms like congestion and itching, or inhale steam with chamomile oil to clear nasal passages. Apply chamomile-infused compresses to reduce eye irritation, or add chamomile to baths to soothe skin reactions.

Mixing chamomile honey into warm drinks can alleviate throat soreness and coughing. Note that individuals allergic to Asteraceae family plants should use chamomile with caution. Consult a healthcare professional before using chamomile, especially if pregnant or nursing.

Incorporating chamomile into your daily routine can naturally support respiratory health and overall well-being by gently managing allergies.

Goldenrod

Goldenrod, often mistaken as an allergy trigger due to its yellow blooms, is actually a powerful ally in allergy management. Rich in anti-inflammatory and antihistamine properties, goldenrod is a valuable natural remedy for easing allergic reactions and respiratory discomfort.

To use goldenrod's anti-allergy effects, brew goldenrod tea or create a tincture from dried flowers to alleviate symptoms like congestion and itchy eyes. Inhaling steam infused with goldenrod essential oil can clear nasal passages, while a saline rinse with goldenrod tincture soothes inflamed mucous membranes. Infusing honey with goldenrod offers a sweet immune boost, while adding goldenrod flowers to baths calms skin irritation and itching.

Caution for individuals allergic to Asteraceae family plants, who may experience cross-reactivity with goldenrod. Consult a healthcare professional before using goldenrod, especially if pregnant or nursing.

HELPING ALL THE FAMILY WITH COUGHS AND COLDS

Respiratory soothers offer gentle relief for coughs and colds in your family. Prepare herbal teas with the following herbs to ease congestion. You may also encourage steam inhalation with eucalyptus oil to immediately relieve stuffiness.

Echinacea

Echinacea, native to North America, boasts purple petals and a cone-shaped center. It's recognized for enhancing the body's immune response against infections, making it a go-to during cold and flu seasons.

With its antiviral and antibacterial properties, echinacea effectively manages coughs and colds by bolstering the immune system. You can harness its respiratory benefits through echinacea tea, supplements (in capsule or liquid form), or homemade remedies like herbal syrups and tinctures crafted from dried echinacea leaves and flowers.

Elderberry

Elderberry, a deep-purple berry from the elder tree, is prized for its robust taste and powerful health benefits. Rich in antioxidants and vitamins, it's particularly valuable during cold and flu season.

Thanks to its immune-boosting properties, elderberry effectively manages coughs and colds. Loaded with flavonoids and anthocyanins, it strengthens the immune system and diminishes the severity and duration of respiratory infections.

To tap into elderberry's respiratory benefits, there are various consumption methods. Elderberry syrup, crafted by simmering elderberries with water and honey or sugar, is a well-loved option. Elderberry supplements, available in syrup or capsule form, provide convenient immune support. Moreover, elderberry tea, brewed with dried berries or tea bags, offers soothing relief for respiratory discomfort.

Eucalyptus

Eucalyptus, a towering evergreen tree native to Australia, is famous for its unique scent and healing properties. Its leaves contain cineole, a compound known for its respiratory benefits.

Eucalyptus effectively manages coughs and colds thanks to its expectorant and decongestant qualities. Inhaling eucalyptus vapors clears the respiratory tract, easing breathing and reducing coughing and congestion.

To experience eucalyptus' respiratory effects, inhalation is key. Add a few drops of eucalyptus oil to hot water and breathe in the steam for congestion relief. Diffuse eucalyptus oil at home or mix it with a carrier oil for chest rubs. Additionally, sipping eucalyptus tea made from dried leaves offers soothing relief for respiratory discomfort.

Marjoram

Marjoram, a delightful herb from the mint family, offers both culinary delights and health benefits. Its gentle aroma and properties make it a favorite in kitchens and remedies alike.

Marjoram is cherished for its role in soothing coughs and managing common cold symptoms. Its compounds effectively ease respiratory issues like congestion and coughing, providing relief during times of discomfort.

To enjoy marjoram's respiratory support, brew it into a comforting tea by steeping dried leaves in hot water. Inhaling the steam infused with marjoram essence can also alleviate nasal congestion and throat irritation. Adding marjoram to soups, stews, or herbal concoctions further amplifies its respiratory-soothing effects when consumed.

PROVEN HERBS FOR CHRONIC RESPIRATORY CONDITIONS

Certain herbs can offer valuable support when dealing with chronic respiratory conditions. Herbs such as mullein, licorice root, and elecampane are known for their ability to help manage symptoms and promote respiratory health. Incorporating these herbs into teas, tinctures, or steam inhalations can relieve and support your respiratory well-being.

Licorice

Licorice, with its sweet taste, holds significant medicinal value. Its roots, containing compounds like glycyrrhizin, offer various health benefits.

Licorice is highly regarded for its capacity to alleviate respiratory discomfort linked to chronic conditions like asthma, bronchitis, and COPD. By reducing inflammation in the respiratory tract and easing coughing, it supports clearer breathing, serving as a valuable aid in managing such issues.

To tap into licorice's respiratory advantages, consider preparing licorice root tea. Licorice root supplements or extracts are also available for herbal remedies. However, it's crucial to use licorice cautiously to avoid potential side effects like elevated blood pressure or potassium depletion.

Always seek advice from a healthcare professional before incorporating licorice into your respiratory regimen, especially if you have existing medical conditions or are taking medications.

Mullein

Mullein, recognized for its tall, fuzzy leaves and bright-yellow flowers, is a renowned herbal remedy for respiratory issues.

It's highly regarded for managing symptoms linked to chronic respiratory conditions like asthma, bronchitis, and COPD. Mullein serves as an expectorant, aiding in mucus loosening and lung congestion relief. Moreover, its anti-inflammatory properties ease respiratory tract inflammation, enhancing breathing and overall lung health.

To benefit from mullein's respiratory advantages, brew mullein tea by steeping dried leaves or flowers in hot water. Regular consumption helps alleviate respiratory discomfort and maintains lung function. Mullein can also be utilized in herbal formulations like tinctures or steam inhalations for targeted respiratory relief. Prior to using mullein, it's advisable to seek advice from a healthcare professional, particularly if you have existing health issues or are on medications.

Ginseng

Ginseng, known for its distinctive forked shape and bright-red berries, holds a revered status in traditional medicine.

Its potent properties support the respiratory system, particularly in chronic conditions like asthma and bronchitis. Ginseng helps improve lung function by relaxing airways and reducing inflammation, thereby enhancing breathing and overall respiratory health.

To harness the benefits of ginseng for respiratory wellness, it can be consumed in various forms such as teas, capsules, or tinctures. Ginseng tea, made from dried ginseng root, is a popular choice for respiratory support. Alternatively, ginseng extracts or supplements can be integrated into daily routines, with guidance from a healthcare professional.

Given potential variations in individual responses to herbal remedies, consult a healthcare provider before incorporating ginseng, especially for those with existing health conditions or who are taking medications.

Wild Cherry

Wild cherry, known for its small red to black cherries and shiny leaves, is a prized North American tree with medicinal value.

Its bark has been traditionally used to ease symptoms of chronic respiratory conditions like coughs, bronchitis, and asthma. Wild cherry bark is thought to have expectorant properties, aiding in mucus loosening and promoting easier breathing, which helps alleviate congestion and coughing.

To benefit from wild cherry's respiratory advantages, the bark can be simmered in water to create a decoction, then consumed as tea. Alternatively, commercially available wild cherry bark extracts or syrups can be used under healthcare professional guidance.

It's important to consult with a healthcare provider before using wild cherry, especially if you have underlying health issues or are on medication, to ensure its suitability and effectiveness for your specific needs.

BREATHE EASY RECIPES

Here are effective solutions for respiratory wellness, primarily through teas, infusions, and steam baths. Herbs known for their respiratory benefits, such as eucalyptus, thyme, and peppermint, soothe and support the respiratory system.

Whether you're seeking relief from congestion or coughing or simply looking to breathe easier, these natural remedies provide gentle and comforting support for your respiratory health.

Stinging Nettle Decoction

This stinging nettle decoction is a powerful remedy for joint pain, combining dried nettle leaves with licorice root for enhanced benefits. Simmer the mixture in water, strain, and enjoy as tea or apply as a compress to sore joints for relief. This natural blend offers holistic joint discomfort management.

Instructions:

1. Bring 2 cups of water to a boil in a saucepan.
2. Add 2 tablespoons of dried stinging nettle leaves and 1 tablespoon of licorice root to the boiling water.

3. Reduce the heat and let the mixture simmer for 10-15 minutes, allowing the herbs to infuse.
4. Remove the saucepan from the heat and let the decoction cool to a comfortable temperature.
5. Strain the mixture using a fine mesh strainer or cheesecloth to remove the herbs.
6. Pour the strained decoction into a mug and sip slowly as a soothing herbal tea.
7. Alternatively, soak a clean cloth in the cooled decoction and apply it as a compress to areas experiencing joint pain for added relief.

Goldenrod and Green Tea

Goldenrod and green tea infusion combines the flavors of goldenrod and green tea, creating a refreshing and invigorating blend with respiratory health benefits. This herbal infusion provides both enjoyment for the palate and natural respiratory support, making it a great choice for those seeking holistic remedies.

Instructions:

1. Boil 2 cups of water in a saucepan and remove it from heat.
2. Add 1 tablespoon of dried goldenrod flowers and 1 green tea bag to the hot water.
3. Cover the saucepan and let the herbs steep for 5-7 minutes, allowing their flavors to infuse into the water.
4. Once steeped, remove the green tea bag and strain the infusion to extract the goldenrod flowers.
5. Pour the infused liquid into a cup and let it cool for a few minutes until it reaches a comfortable drinking temperature.

6. Sip the goldenrod and green tea infusion slowly, enjoying its soothing taste and respiratory benefits.
7. For added sweetness, you may stir in a teaspoon of honey if desired.
8. Relax and indulge in this comforting herbal blend, knowing it's providing nourishment and support for your lungs and overall well-being.

Peppermint and Eucalyptus Steam Bath

Revitalize with a peppermint and eucalyptus steam bath, perfect for clearing congestion and refreshing your respiratory system. Add rosemary for extra therapeutic benefits. Fresh ingredients guarantee optimal potency, ensuring a rejuvenating experience.

Instructions:

1. Boil a pot of water on the stove until it reaches a rolling boil.
2. Once boiling, remove the pot and transfer the hot water to a heat-safe bowl or basin.
3. Add a handful of fresh peppermint, eucalyptus, and rosemary sprigs to the hot water.
4. Allow the aromatic herbs to steep in the water for a few minutes, releasing their soothing vapors.
5. Position your face over the bowl, ensuring a safe distance to avoid burns, and drape a towel over your head to trap the steam.
6. Close your eyes and inhale deeply, allowing the invigorating steam to penetrate your airways and soothe congestion.
7. Take slow, deep breaths for 5-10 minutes, allowing the herbal steam to work its magic.

8. After the steam session, pat your face dry with a clean towel and rinse with cool water to close your pores.
9. Enjoy the refreshing sensation and the clear breathing that follows, knowing you've treated your respiratory system to a revitalizing experience.

Ginseng Tea

Elevate your day with a revitalizing Ginseng Tea, renowned for its energizing properties and potential health benefits. This refreshing beverage significantly boosts your energy levels and overall well-being.

Instructions:

1. Start by bringing water to a gentle boil in a saucepan or kettle.
2. While the water heats, thoroughly prepare your ginseng root under cold water to remove dirt or debris.
3. Use a sharp knife to thinly slice the ginseng root into small pieces, increasing the surface area for optimal infusion.
4. Once the water reaches a boil, reduce the heat to a simmer and add the sliced ginseng root to the pot.
5. Allow the ginseng to steep in the simmering water for approximately 15-20 minutes, allowing its essence to infuse into the liquid.
6. Consider adding a slice of fresh ginger or a dash of honey to the tea for added flavor and health benefits.
7. After steeping, remove the pot from the heat and strain the tea to remove the ginseng root pieces.
8. Pour the freshly brewed ginseng tea into your favorite mug and savor the refreshing aroma and flavor.

9. Take a moment to enjoy your ginseng tea and embrace the natural energy and vitality it brings to your day.

Mullein and Thyme Tea

Enjoy mullein and thyme tea for its soothing and respiratory-supporting qualities. This comforting blend combines mullein's gentleness with thyme's aromatic essence, creating a calming and supportive beverage for your respiratory wellness.

Instructions:

1. Begin by boiling water in a saucepan or kettle until it reaches a gentle simmer.
2. While the water heats, prepare your herbs in cold water to remove impurities.
3. Measure out approximately 1-2 teaspoons of dried mullein leaves and 1 teaspoon of dried thyme leaves for each cup of tea you plan to brew.
4. Once the water reaches a simmer, add the dried mullein and thyme leaves to the pot.
5. Allow the herbs to steep in the simmering water for 10-15 minutes, releasing their beneficial compounds and flavors.
6. Consider adding a spoonful of honey or a slice of lemon to your tea for added sweetness or flavor.
7. After steeping, remove the pot from the heat and strain the tea to remove the herb leaves.
8. Pour the freshly brewed mullein and thyme tea into your favorite mug, inhaling its soothing aroma.
9. Take a moment to sip and enjoy the comforting warmth and herbal goodness of your mullein and thyme tea, embracing its supportive properties for respiratory health.

Peppermint, Elderberry, and Mullein Infusion

Experience the refreshing and immune-boosting peppermint, elderberry, and mullein infusion. This blend combines peppermint's invigorating essence, elderberry's immune support, and mullein's soothing effects for a delicious and beneficial beverage.

Instructions:

1. Begin by boiling water in a saucepan or kettle until it reaches a gentle simmer.
2. While the water heats, prepare your herbs in cold water to remove impurities.
3. Measure out approximately 1-2 teaspoons of dried peppermint leaves, 1 teaspoon of dried elderberries, and 1 teaspoon of dried mullein leaves for each cup of infusion you plan to brew.
4. Once the water reaches a simmer, add the dried peppermint, elderberries, and mullein leaves to the pot.
5. Allow the herbs to steep in the simmering water for 10-15 minutes, allowing their flavors and beneficial compounds to infuse into the water.
6. After steeping, remove the pot from the heat and strain the infusion to remove the herb leaves and berries.
7. Pour the freshly brewed peppermint, elderberry, and mullein infusion into your favorite mug or teapot, admiring its vibrant color and refreshing aroma.
8. Take a moment to savor each sip of this nourishing infusion, embracing its immune-boosting properties and refreshing taste.

Licorice, Lavender, and Chamomile Tea

Enjoy the soothing licorice, lavender, and chamomile tea, perfect for relaxing your mind and body. This delightful blend offers the gentle sweetness of licorice root, paired with the floral notes of lavender and the calming essence of chamomile.

Instructions:

1. Begin by boiling fresh water in a kettle or saucepan until it reaches a rolling boil.
2. While the water heats, gather your herbs, ensuring they are clean and debris-free.
3. Measure out approximately 1-2 teaspoons of dried licorice root, 1 teaspoon of dried lavender flowers, and 1 teaspoon of dried chamomile flowers per cup of tea you plan to brew.
4. Once the water reaches a boil, remove it from the heat and pour it over the measured herbs in a teapot or heat-resistant container.
5. Cover the teapot or container with a lid or plate to trap the steam and allow the herbs to steep for 5-10 minutes.
6. After steeping, strain the tea into your favorite cup or mug, using a fine mesh strainer or tea infuser to remove the herb particles.
7. Take a moment to inhale the soothing aroma of the licorice, lavender, and chamomile tea, allowing its fragrance to calm your senses.
8. Sip slowly and enjoy this comforting herbal blend's gentle sweetness and floral notes, letting it ease your tensions and promote relaxation.

Elderberry, Echinacea, and Wild Cherry Syrup

Savor the potent elderberry, echinacea, and wild cherry syrup, crafted to boost your immune system and ease seasonal discomfort. This blend combines the immune-strengthening properties of elderberry and echinacea with the soothing effects of wild cherry, offering relief from cold and flu symptoms.

Instructions:

1. Begin by gathering the necessary ingredients: dried elderberries, dried echinacea root or herb, dried wild cherry bark, water, and honey.
2. In a saucepan, combine 1 cup of dried elderberries, 2 tablespoons of dried echinacea root or herb, and 2 tablespoons of dried wild cherry bark with 4 cups of water.
3. Bring the mixture to a gentle boil over medium heat, then reduce the heat and let it simmer uncovered for about 30-45 minutes, or until the liquid is reduced by half.
4. Once the liquid has reduced, remove the saucepan from the heat and allow the mixture to cool slightly.
5. Strain the liquid through a fine mesh strainer or cheesecloth into a clean bowl or measuring cup, pressing down on the herbs to extract as much liquid as possible.
6. Once strained, return the liquid to the saucepan and place it on the stove over low heat.
7. Gradually stir in honey to taste, starting with about 1/2 to 1 cup of honey for sweetness and added immune support.
8. Continue to heat the mixture gently, stirring constantly, until the honey dissolves and the syrup is well combined.

9. Remove the syrup from the heat and let it cool completely before transferring it to a clean, airtight glass jar or bottle for storage.
10. Store the elderberry, echinacea, and wild cherry syrup in the refrigerator for up to 2-3 months, and take as needed to support your immune system and soothe respiratory symptoms during cold and flu season.

CONCLUSION

There is one other organ that can't be forgotten in the quest for herbal healing. As we move on to the B in the HERBS method, we will next discover how to keep the brain in optimal health, whether you are studying for an exam or reducing the risk of debilitating neurological conditions. Get ready for Brain Boosters in Chapter 7.

B: BRAIN BOOSTERS

Herbal remedies are not just good for common ailments. Many herbs are brain boosters; simple herbs found in your spice rack can enhance focus, concentration, and cognitive function.

This chapter is about the remarkable properties of herbs and spices that nourish and support the brain, offering insights into how they can combat neurocognitive impairments such as dementia.

Do you know that the brain is the body's most voracious organ, consuming significant energy? This is why you must provide the brain with the nutrients it craves for optimal function and long-term health.

WHAT OXIDATIVE STRESS AND INFLAMMATION IS DOING TO YOUR BRAIN

Oxidative stress and inflammation are major threats to brain health, hastening cognitive decline and raising the risk of neurodegenerative diseases like Alzheimer's and Parkinson's. With dementia affecting millions globally and its prevalence set to increase, understanding these processes is crucial.

Medicinal plants offer promising remedies, reducing the risk and slowing down disease progression. Surprisingly, research suggests one in three dementia cases is preventable, highlighting the potential for proactive measures and natural remedies to protect brain health (Kales, 2017).

Taking proactive steps not only reduces the risk of chronic conditions but also enhances focus, enabling us to tackle mental tasks efficiently and boost overall cognitive performance.

BRAIN FOG NO MORE

Herbal brain boosters can remarkably clear up brain fog, restoring mental clarity and sharpness. They enhance cognitive function, improve memory, and promote mental alertness.

Incorporating these herbal remedies into your daily routine can help you overcome brain fog and optimize your brain health for better productivity and overall well-being.

Sage

Sage, a fragrant herb with gray-green leaves, boasts ancient medicinal benefits and is now cultivated worldwide. It's revered for its ability to enhance cognitive function, memory, and focus. Compounds like rosmarinic acid and carnosic acid in sage provide antioxidant and anti-inflammatory properties, promoting brain health by safeguarding brain cells.

To harness sage's anti-brain fog effects, integrate it into your daily routine. Make sage tea by steeping fresh or dried leaves, or add fresh sage to soups, stews, and salads for its unique flavor and cognitive benefits. Sage supplements, available in capsules or extracts, offer convenient cognitive support.

Bacopa

Bacopa, also known as brahmi, is a small herb native to wetlands in India, Australia, and Europe, prized for its medicinal benefits in Ayurvedic medicine. It's celebrated for improving memory, learning, and cognitive function due to its bacosides, active compounds that support brain neurotransmitters.

Bacopa's antioxidants also protect brain cells from oxidative stress, potentially slowing cognitive decline with age. Add bacopa into your routine through supplements or by brewing bacopa tea from dried leaves for a soothing beverage. Consult a healthcare professional before adding new herbal supplements to your routine.

Rosemary

Rosemary, scientifically known as Rosmarinus officinalis, is a fragrant herb from the Mediterranean region, prized globally for its culinary and medicinal uses. Its slender leaves and blue flowers emit a pine-like scent.

Rosemary enhances cognitive function, memory, and mental clarity, with its aroma linked to improved mood and concentration. Compounds like carnosic acid in rosemary have neuroprotective effects, potentially preventing age-related cognitive decline.

Incorporate rosemary into your routine by brewing tea or infusing it into olive oil for cooking.

Besides its scent, rosemary's ability to boost circulation promotes mental well-being. Whether in cooking or aromatherapy, rosemary offers a natural solution to combat brain fog and enhance cognitive function.

Lion's Mane

Lion's Mane, scientifically known as Hericium erinaceus, is a unique mushroom with a shaggy appearance resembling a lion's mane. Found in North America, Europe, and Asia, it's valued in traditional medicine.

This mushroom supports cognitive function and mental clarity. Compounds like hericenones and erinacines may stimulate nerve growth factor (NGF) production, enhancing brain health. It's believed to alleviate brain fog and mental fatigue.

Include lion's mane in your diet or as a supplement in various forms like fresh, dried, or extract. It's versatile, adding to soups, stir-fries, and teas. Supplements in capsule or powder form offer convenient consumption, potentially improving cognitive function and focus naturally.

Peppermint

Peppermint, or Mentha piperita, is a well-known herb cherished for its refreshing scent and taste. Originating from Europe and Asia, its vibrant green leaves emit a minty fragrance.

Peppermint is valued for its ability to improve cognitive function and mental clarity. Its menthol compounds are linked to heightened alertness, focus, and memory retention.

The scent of peppermint can also reduce mental fatigue and increase wakefulness.

Integrate peppermint into your daily routine for its anti-brain fog effects. Enjoy peppermint tea or inhale its essential oil for mental alertness. Use it in cooking, beverages, and home remedies to enhance flavors and boost vitality. Whether in tea, aromatherapy, or cooking, peppermint offers a natural way to refresh your mind and enhance cognitive function.

NEUROPROTECTIVE HERBS AND SPICES

Neuroprotective herbs and spices support and protect the health of the brain and nervous system. These natural remedies offer potential benefits for cognitive function, memory retention, and overall brain health.

Including neuroprotective herbs and spices in your diet and lifestyle can help enhance brain function and reduce the risk of neurodegenerative conditions. Explore the power of these natural remedies to safeguard your brain health and promote overall well-being.

Gotu Kola

Gotu kola, also known as Centella asiatica, is a small plant native to Asia, prized in Ayurvedic and traditional Chinese medicine. It has fan-shaped leaves and small white or pink flowers.

Gotu kola offers neuroprotective benefits that enhance brain health and cognitive function. Compounds like asiaticoside and Asiatic acid improve memory, reduce oxidative stress, and boost brain circulation.

You can enjoy gotu kola in teas, extracts, capsules, or fresh in salads. Adding gotu kola to your daily routine may support mental clarity, focus, and overall brain function.

Ashwagandha

Ashwagandha, also called Withania somnifera, is a well-known adaptogenic herb from India, the Middle East, and parts of Africa. It's a small shrub with yellow flowers and valuable roots and leaves.

Ashwagandha offers strong neuroprotective benefits due to compounds like withanolides and alkaloids. These fight inflammation, oxidative stress, and brain amyloid beta buildup, improving cognitive function and guarding against Alzheimer's and Parkinson's.

You can find Ashwagandha in capsules, powders, teas, or tinctures. Regular use may enhance memory, focus, and overall brain health, helping you better handle stress.

Saffron

Saffron, from the Crocus sativus flower, is prized for its red color and unique flavor. Its aroma and medicinal properties make it popular worldwide.

Saffron has strong neuroprotective qualities due to compounds like crocin, crocetin, and safranal. Research shows they have antioxidant and anti-inflammatory effects, which may help with conditions like Alzheimer's and Parkinson's.

You can use saffron in cooking, teas, or supplements. Regular intake may improve cognitive abilities and reduce brain oxidative stress. However, consult a healthcare professional before using saffron for Alzheimer's or Parkinson's. Growing saffron at home is an option to consider.

Ginkgo Biloba

Ginkgo biloba, known as the maidenhair tree, is valued in Chinese medicine for its leaves and aroma. It's praised for its potential to improve brain health and cognitive function.

Ginkgo biloba has antioxidants that shield nerve cells.

These compounds enhance brain blood flow, support brain flexibility, and improve neurotransmitter function, which may enhance memory and cognition. Studies suggest it could also prevent age-related cognitive decline and Alzheimer's.

Ginkgo biloba supplements come in various strengths. Taking them daily may boost cognitive function and memory and lower the risk of cognitive decline. However, consult a healthcare professional before starting any new supplements, especially if you have medical conditions or take medications.

Moringa

Moringa, from Africa and Asia, is prized for its nutrients and health perks. Its leaves, seeds, and pods are loaded with vitamins, minerals, and antioxidants, making it a dietary gem.

Rich in antioxidants like flavonoids and vitamin C, moringa fights brain inflammation and stress.

These substances keep nerve cells healthy, lower neurodegenerative disease risk, and enhance memory and cognition. Studies suggest moringa may combat Alzheimer's, Parkinson's, and age-related cognitive decline.

Adding moringa to meals is simple. Fresh, dried, or powdered leaves blend well in smoothies, salads, soups, and stir-fries for added nutrition. Moringa supplements in capsules, powders, or extracts offer convenience. Opt for trusted sources and consult a healthcare expert before trying it, especially if you have health concerns or are pregnant or breastfeeding.

SIMPLE RECIPES TO FUEL YOUR BRAIN

Brain-boosting herbal remedies in your daily diet can enhance cognitive function, improve focus, and support overall brain health. Whether you're looking to clear brain fog, enhance memory, or protect against neurological conditions, these simple recipes offer a delicious way to fuel your brain.

Moringa and Peppermint Tea

Moringa, a superfood rich in nutrients, combines with the refreshing taste of peppermint in this invigorating tea. The earthy notes of moringa are balanced by peppermint's cool, minty flavor, creating a revitalizing blend that's both nutritious and refreshing.

Instructions:

1. Boil water in a kettle or pot.
2. Place a teaspoon of dried moringa leaves and a few fresh peppermint leaves in a teapot or heatproof mug.
3. Pour the hot water over the leaves.
4. Let the tea steep for 5-7 minutes to allow the flavors to infuse fully.
5. Add a squeeze of fresh lemon juice and a drizzle of honey to enhance the flavor.
6. Strain the tea into cups and enjoy the rejuvenating goodness of moringa and peppermint.

Lion's Mane, Cardamon, Ginger, and Cinnamon Tea

Indulge in the warm and comforting flavors of lion's mane, cardamom, ginger, and cinnamon tea. This aromatic blend delights the senses and offers a nourishing boost to your mind and body, making it the perfect beverage to start your day or unwind in the evening.

Instructions:

1. Bring water to a boil in a pot or kettle.
2. Add a few slices of fresh ginger, a couple of crushed cardamom pods, a pinch of cinnamon powder, and a

teaspoon of dried lion's mane mushroom to a teapot or heatproof mug.
3. Pour the hot water over the ingredients in the teapot or mug.
4. Allow the tea to steep for 7-10 minutes to infuse the flavors thoroughly.
5. Strain the tea into cups to remove the solid ingredients.
6. Optionally, add a touch of honey or a splash of milk for sweetness and creaminess.
7. Savor the rich flavors and rejuvenating properties of lion's mane, cardamom, ginger, and cinnamon tea.

Rosemary and Sage Infusion

Experience the refreshing blend of rosemary and sage infusion, awakening your senses and revitalizing your mind. This infusion combines earthy and aromatic flavors, ideal for enjoying as a tea or using in aromatherapy diffusers to invigorate your senses with rejuvenating scents.

Instructions:

1. Boil water in a pot or kettle.
2. Meanwhile, gather fresh rosemary sprigs and sage leaves, rinsing them thoroughly under cold water.
3. Place the washed herbs in a teapot or heatproof mug.
4. Once the water boils, pour it over the herbs in the teapot or mug.
5. Allow the herbs to steep in the hot water for about 5-10 minutes, depending on your desired strength of flavor.
6. Strain the infusion into cups to remove the herbs.
7. Enjoy the aromatic and flavorful rosemary and sage infusion as a soothing tea, or add it to aromatherapy

diffusers for a fragrant and refreshing inhalation experience.

Ashwaganda Tincture

Utilize ashwagandha's adaptogenic power with a homemade tincture. Also called Indian ginseng, ashwagandha is esteemed for stress relief and holistic health. Crafting your ashwagandha tincture enables seamless integration into your daily regimen, supporting vitality and resilience.

Instructions:

1. Begin by obtaining high-quality ashwagandha root or powder from a trusted source.
2. If using dried ashwagandha root, finely chop or grind it to increase surface area and facilitate extraction.
3. Combine the chopped or powdered ashwagandha in a clean glass jar with a suitable menstruum, such as high-proof vodka or grain alcohol. The ratio of herb to alcohol typically ranges from 1:2 to 1:5, depending on the desired potency.
4. Ensure the ashwagandha is fully submerged in the alcohol, and tightly seal the jar.
5. Store the jar in a cool, dark place, gently shaking it every day to promote thorough extraction.
6. Allow the mixture to steep for at least 4-6 weeks, allowing the alcohol to extract the beneficial compounds from the ashwagandha.
7. After the steeping period, strain the tincture through a fine mesh strainer or cheesecloth into a clean glass bottle, pressing out as much liquid as possible from the herb material.

8. Label the bottle with the date and contents, and store it in a cool, dark place for long-term storage.
9. Take the desired dosage of ashwagandha tincture as recommended by a qualified herbalist or healthcare practitioner, either directly under the tongue or diluted in a small amount of water or juice.

Infused Vinegar and Oil With Ginkgo Biloba, Bacopa, and Gotu Kola

Elevate your dishes with an infused vinegar and oil recipe featuring brain-boosting herbs like ginkgo biloba, bacopa, and gotu kola. This infusion not only enhances flavor but also promotes health. Including these herbs into your daily meals supports cognitive function and overall well-being.

Instructions:

1. Gather fresh or dried ginkgo biloba, bacopa, and gotu kola leaves or powder from a reputable source.
2. Thoroughly wash and dry the herbs to remove any dirt or impurities.
3. Place the desired combination of herbs in separate glass jars for each infusion. You can experiment with different ratios based on your taste preferences.
4. Fill each jar with high-quality vinegar or oil, ensuring that the herbs are completely submerged.
5. Seal the jars tightly with lids and store them in a cool, dark place away from direct sunlight.
6. Allow the herbs to infuse into the vinegar and oil for at least 2-4 weeks, shaking the jars gently every few days to encourage extraction.

7. After the infusion, strain the vinegar and oil through a fine mesh strainer or cheesecloth into clean glass bottles, pressing out any excess liquid from the herbs.
8. Label the bottles with the date and contents, and store them in the refrigerator to prolong shelf life and preserve freshness.
9. Use the infused vinegar to add a flavorful twist to salads, dressings, and sauces, while the infused oil can be drizzled over vegetables, pasta, or bread for an aromatic touch.
10. Enjoy the delicious taste and brain-boosting benefits of your homemade infused vinegar and oil creations in your everyday culinary adventures.

Saffron Milk

Saffron milk is a golden elixir known for its rich flavor and medicinal perks. Its aroma and taste delight the senses, while its skin-nourishing qualities promote overall well-being. Incorporating saffron milk into your daily routine fosters self-care and nurtures radiant skin from within.

Instructions:

1. Begin by gathering high-quality saffron threads and fresh milk. Opt for organic or locally sourced ingredients for the best flavor and nutritional value.
2. Heat the desired amount of milk in a saucepan over medium heat until it simulates gently. Avoid boiling the milk, as this can alter its taste and texture.
3. While the milk is heating, crush a few strands of saffron between your fingertips to release its aromatic compounds and vibrant color.

4. Once the milk is warm, add the crushed saffron strands to the saucepan and gently stir to distribute the saffron evenly.
5. Allow the saffron-infused milk to simmer gently for 5-7 minutes, allowing the flavors to meld and the saffron to infuse into the milk.
6. Remove the saucepan from the heat and let the saffron milk cool slightly before serving.
7. Pour the saffron milk into a cup or mug, using a fine mesh strainer to remove any remaining saffron strands if desired.
8. Savor the aromatic and velvety-smooth saffron milk as a soothing bedtime beverage or a midday treat for relaxation and rejuvenation.
9. For an added skin-nourishing boost, apply a small amount of saffron milk topically to your skin, gently massaging it to promote hydration and a radiant complexion.
10. Incorporate saffron milk into your daily self-care routine to indulge in its exquisite flavor and experience the transformative benefits it offers for your skin and overall well-being.

Lion's Mane and Bacopa Coffee

Boost your morning routine with lion's mane and bacopa-infused coffee, a unique blend that enhances cognitive function and tantalizes your taste buds. Experience the rich flavors and refreshing benefits of this synergistic combination, giving you a focused and refreshing start to your day.

Instructions:

1. Brew your favorite coffee using your preferred method, ensuring it reaches your desired strength and flavor profile.
2. Gather lion's mane and bacopa powder from your local health food store or online supplier as your coffee brews.
3. Once your coffee is ready, pour it into your favorite mug or cup.
4. Add a pinch of lion's mane and bacopa powder to your freshly brewed coffee. Begin with a small amount and adjust according to your taste preferences.
5. Use a spoon or stirrer to thoroughly mix the powders into your coffee, ensuring they blend evenly.
6. Take a moment to savor the enticing aroma and rich flavors of lion's mane and bacopa-infused coffee.
7. Experiment with different ratios of lion's Mane, bacopa, and coffee to find the perfect balance that suits your taste and desired cognitive benefits.
8. Consider adding complementary ingredients like saffron milk to enhance your coffee's flavor profile and nourishing properties.
9. Incorporate lion's mane and bacopa coffee into your daily routine for a refreshing and focused start to your day, harnessing the cognitive-enhancing effects of these powerful herbs.
10. Enjoy each sip of your lion's mane and bacopa-infused coffee, knowing you're fueling your mind and body with revitalizing nutrients and delicious flavors.

Sage, Rosemary, and Moringa Tincture

Creating a tincture with sage, rosemary, and moringa offers a potent blend for enhancing concentration and protecting the mind and body. Remember, when preparing this tincture, avoid using powdered herbs as they may result in a less effective extraction process.

Instructions:

1. **Gather Your Ingredients**: Obtain fresh sage leaves, rosemary sprigs, and moringa leaves from a reputable source. Ensure the herbs are thoroughly cleaned and free from any dirt or debris.
2. **Select Your Base Alcohol**: Choose a high-proof alcohol such as vodka or brandy for optimal extraction of the herbs' beneficial compounds. The alcohol acts as a solvent, extracting the active ingredients from the herbs.
3. **Prepare Your Jar**: Use a clean, sterilized glass jar with an airtight lid to hold your tincture. Ensure the jar is large enough to accommodate the herbs and alcohol while leaving some space at the top for shaking and mixing.
4. **Combine the Herbs and Alcohol**: Fill the glass jar with sage leaves, rosemary sprigs, and moringa leaves, ensuring they are loosely packed for proper extraction. Pour the alcohol over the herbs, covering them completely.
5. **Seal and Shake**: Secure the lid tightly on the jar and give it a good shake to ensure the herbs are evenly distributed and submerged in the alcohol. Label the jar with the date of preparation and the contents.
6. **Steep and Store**: Place the jar in a cool, dark place away from direct sunlight. Allow the herbs to steep in the alcohol for at least 4-6 weeks, shaking the jar gently every few days to promote thorough extraction.
7. **Strain and Bottle**: After steeping, strain the tincture through a fine mesh strainer or cheesecloth into a clean glass bottle. Squeeze out any excess liquid from the herbs to extract all the tincture's goodness.

8. **Store and Enjoy**: Transfer the strained tincture into amber glass bottles with dropper caps for convenient storage and use. Store the bottles in a cool, dark place, and use the tincture as needed to support concentration and overall well-being.

Following these simple steps, you can create a potent sage, rosemary, and moringa tincture to enhance your focus and promote mental clarity and protection. Consult with a healthcare professional before incorporating new herbal remedies into your wellness routine.

CONCLUSION

The first four steps of the HERBS framework have focused on physical health. Despite having benefits on mental well-being, the final step will focus more on reducing the impact and symptoms of stress, anxiety, and depression, three conditions that are all too common nowadays! See you in Stress Relievers in Chapter 8.

S: STRESS RELIEVERS

"Stress is the trash of modern life. We all generate it, but if you don't dispose of it properly, it will pile up and overtake your life." –Danzae Pace

Stress can wreak havoc on your body and mind if left unchecked. It isn't something you must accept as normal—you must manage and overcome it.

Inspired by Danzae Pace's wise words, this chapter confronts stress head-on. Just like piling up trash, it can overwhelm you if you don't deal with stress properly. However, amid the chaos, you can rely on the healing power of nature's remedies called stress relievers.

Let us explore how herbal remedies can offer relief from the burdens of stress, anxiety, and depression, providing a sanctuary for your weary soul.

Let's uncover the soothing properties of various herbs. From ancient traditions to modern insights, these plants hold the key to restoring balance and tranquility to your life. Find new ways to nourish your body, calm your mind, and reclaim your inner peace.

IT'S TIME TO BEAT THAT STRESS

Stress affects more than just your mind—it impacts your entire body, including your gut health. The brain-gut axis, connecting your brain and digestive system, is sensitive to stress. When stress strikes, it disrupts this balance, leading to digestive issues like bloating and irritable bowel syndrome (IBS).

Recognizing the link between stress and digestion is crucial. By understanding how stress influences your gut, you can take steps to restore balance and regain control over your well-being.

OPTIMAL HERBS FOR STRESS, ANXIETY, AND DEPRESSION

Optimal herbal remedies for natural relief of stress, anxiety, and depression work by soothing the nervous system and promoting relaxation. They work synergistically with the body to restore balance and calm the mind, helping alleviate emotional distress symptoms.

Including these herbs in your daily routine can provide a holistic approach to managing stress and improving overall mental well-being.

Holy Basil

Holy basil, also known as tulsi, is a revered herb in Ayurvedic medicine, cherished for its aromatic leaves and unique flavor. It possesses adaptogenic properties, which help the body manage stress and build resilience. By regulating stress hormones like cortisol, it reduces anxiety and induces a sense of calm.

Enjoy holy basil as tea, tincture, or in culinary dishes. Sipping holy basil tea daily or adding fresh leaves to salads and smoothies are popular methods to experience its stress-relieving benefits. Holy basil supplements are also available for convenient stress management.

Ashwagandha

Ashwagandha, also known as Indian ginseng or winter cherry, holds a significant place in traditional Ayurvedic medicine, originating from India. Its name "ashwagandha" in Sanskrit means "smell of the horse," highlighting its distinctive aroma and historical association with vitality and strength.

It acts as an adaptogen, aiding the body in adapting to stress and maintaining balance. By reducing cortisol levels, the primary stress hormone, it fosters relaxation and eases anxiety. Consistent use of ashwagandha may bolster resilience to stressors and enhance overall well-being.

Ashwagandha is available in capsules, powders, and tinctures for easy consumption. It can also be infused into teas or added to beverages like smoothies. Starting with a modest dose and gradually adjusting is advisable to gauge individual response. Consulting a healthcare professional is prudent, especially for those with medical conditions or taking medications.

Skullcap

Skullcap, a perennial herb in the mint family, is known for its delicate blue flowers and helmet-shaped seed pods. Indigenous to North America, it has a long history in traditional herbal medicine, with Scutellaria lateriflora and Scutellaria baicalensis being commonly used.

This herb has calming qualities, providing relief from stress and promoting relaxation. Its flavonoids like baicalin and wogonin are believed to ease anxiety by affecting neurotransmitters. Skullcap is often used to soothe nervous tension, encourage restful sleep, and enhance emotional well-being.

Make skullcap tea by steeping dried leaves and flowers in hot water for 10-15 minutes. Sip this tea throughout the day to reduce stress and induce relaxation. Alternatively, skullcap is available in tinctures and capsules for different preferences.

Begin with a low dose and adjust gradually while monitoring your body's response. Consulting a healthcare professional is wise, particularly if you have health concerns or take medications.

Linden

Linden, also known as tilia or lime flower, is a flowering tree native to Europe and North America. Its fragrant, yellow-white flowers are popular in herbal teas and remedies, adding ornamental beauty to parks and gardens.

Linden offers calming and soothing effects that help manage stress, anxiety, and depression. Its flowers contain compounds like flavonoids and volatile oils, which relax the nervous system and promote tranquility. Additionally, linden's analgesic properties can relieve pain, reducing stress and anxiety.

Enjoy its stress-relieving benefits by steeping dried flowers in hot water for 5-10 minutes to make herbal tea. Sip this tea throughout the day, especially during stressful times. For added relaxation, mix linden with other calming herbs like chamomile or lemon balm. Adding linden tea to your daily routine supports emotional balance and overall well-being.

Kava Kava

Kava kava, also known as Piper methysticum, originates from the South Pacific islands. Its roots are used to create a calming drink in traditional ceremonies. It's valued for its ability to induce relaxation and has been part of cultural rituals for centuries.

This herb contains kavalactones, which interact with brain neurotransmitters to reduce anxiety and promote relaxation. Many use it as a natural stress-relief option.

To benefit from kava kava, make a decoction or tincture from the root. Extract its compounds using water or alcohol. Use kava kava cautiously and consult a healthcare professional before trying it, especially if you have health issues or take medications.

Passionflower

Passionflower, scientifically called Passiflora incarnata, is a climbing vine found in the southeastern United States. Its beautiful flowers and foliage make it a popular ornamental plant, but it's also valued in herbal medicine for its calming effects.

Passionflower is known for its ability to reduce stress and anxiety. It contains compounds like flavonoids and alkaloids that gently calm the nervous system, promoting relaxation. People often use passionflower to ease symptoms of anxiety, insomnia, and nervousness.

To enjoy the stress-relieving benefits of passionflower, brew a calming tea or tincture using the plant's leaves, stems, and flowers. Steep dried passionflower in hot water for a few minutes to create a soothing herbal drink. Alternatively, take passionflower tinctures orally for convenient stress relief.

Before adding passionflower to your routine, consult a healthcare professional, especially if you're pregnant, nursing, or taking medications.

CALMING YOUR DIGESTIVE SYSTEM

Herbal remedies can offer soothing relief. Using stress-relieving herbs in your routine can help calm digestive discomfort and promote overall gut health. These natural remedies can be enjoyed as teas, infusions, or tinctures, offering gentle support for your digestive system during stress.

Cinnamon

Cinnamon is a spice known for its sweet taste and delightful aroma, derived from the inner bark of certain trees. It has natural properties that can soothe the digestive system, potentially reducing bloating, gas, and indigestion discomfort.

To benefit from cinnamon's digestive relief, add a pinch of ground cinnamon to your meals, smoothies, or teas daily. Alternatively, steep cinnamon sticks in hot water for a comforting post-meal drink. Cinnamon capsules or tinctures offer a more concentrated option.

Fennel

Fennel is a fragrant herb with feathery leaves and a mild licorice flavor, commonly used in Mediterranean dishes. It soothes the digestive system by relaxing gastrointestinal muscles, easing bloating, gas, and cramps, thanks to compounds like anethole.

To benefit from fennel's digestive support, chew on its seeds after meals to aid digestion and freshen breath. Brew fennel tea by steeping crushed seeds in hot water, or add chopped fennel bulbs to salads, soups, or stir-fries for added flavor and digestive comfort.

Peppermint

Peppermint is a well-known herb cherished for its cooling taste and invigorating scent. With serrated leaves and small flowers, it's a staple in culinary and herbal practices. Peppermint contains menthol, a natural compound that calms the digestive system. It eases indigestion, bloating, and stomach discomfort by relaxing gastrointestinal muscles and encouraging bile flow.

Enjoy peppermint tea to soothe an upset stomach and aid digestion. Peppermint oil capsules offer a convenient way to relieve digestive issues. You can also add fresh or dried peppermint leaves to salads, smoothies, or infused water for a refreshing and digestive-friendly touch to your meals.

Oregano

Oregano, a fragrant herb in the mint family, is a staple in Mediterranean cuisine and herbal medicine. Its small, oval leaves boast a strong aroma and flavor, enhancing various dishes like pasta and sauces.

Oregano contains carvacrol and thymol, compounds known for their antimicrobial and anti-inflammatory properties. These qualities soothe the digestive system, easing discomfort and promoting gut health by fighting inflammation and harmful bacteria.

Incorporate oregano into your meals by adding fresh or dried leaves to soups, salads, and roasted veggies for aromatic flavor and digestive benefits. Enjoy oregano tea by steeping its leaves in hot water. Oregano essential oil, diluted and used with guidance, can offer targeted digestive support, both internally and topically.

Aloe Vera

Aloe vera, a succulent plant with thick, fleshy leaves, is renowned for its gel-like substance. Originating from tropical climates, it's long been utilized in traditional medicine and skincare. Its leaves are elongated with serrated edges, making it suitable for both indoor and outdoor cultivation.

Aloe vera gel is comprised of polysaccharides, vitamins, minerals, and amino acids, contributing to its gut-calming qualities. Known for its soothing effects, it aids in relieving indigestion, heartburn, and occasional digestive discomfort. Its gentle nature supports gut health and regularity.

To benefit from aloe vera's digestive relief, incorporate its gel into your diet or skincare routine. Extract fresh gel from the leaves, consume it as juice, or add it to smoothies. Topically, aloe vera gel can soothe skin irritation and aid healing. Always ensure purity and consult a healthcare professional, especially if pregnant or with health concerns, before internal use.

Flaxseed

Flaxseed, also known as linseed, is prized for its nutritional benefits. These small seeds are rich in essential fatty acids, fiber, and nutrients. They can calm the gut, thanks to their soluble fiber content. This fiber absorbs water in the digestive tract, forming a gel-like substance that regulates bowel movements and supports digestive health.

Incorporate flaxseed into your daily diet by adding ground flaxseed to smoothies, yogurt, oatmeal, or baked goods. You can also use flaxseed oil in salads or as a topping for dishes to boost nutrition. Drink plenty of water when consuming flaxseed to aid digestion and prevent discomfort. Start with small amounts and gradually increase intake for optimal digestive relief.

TEAS, TINCTURES, AND CULINARY USES OF HERBS FOR STRESS AND DIGESTION

Let us explore a variety of recipes that use herbs known for their stress-relieving properties and digestive benefits. From soothing teas to potent tinctures and creative culinary uses, these recipes offer holistic approaches to promote relaxation and support optimal digestion.

Passionflower, Valerian, and Lemon Balm Tea

Passionflower, valerian, and lemon balm tea is a calming blend that helps alleviate stress and promote relaxation.

Instructions:

1. Boil the water in a small pot.
2. Add the dried passionflower, valerian root, and lemon balm to the boiling water.
3. Reduce the heat and let the herbs simmer for 10-15 minutes.
4. Strain the tea into a cup and let it cool slightly before drinking.
5. Enjoy your calming and soothing passionflower, valerian, and lemon balm tea!

Skullcap, Holy Basil, and Chamomile Tea

Skullcap, holy basil, and chamomile tea is a soothing blend known for its stress-relieving properties and potential to alleviate headaches and aid digestion.

Instructions:

1. Boil the water in a small pot.
2. Add the dried skullcap, holy basil, and chamomile to the boiling water.
3. Reduce the heat and let the herbs simmer for 10-15 minutes.
4. Strain the tea into a cup and cool slightly before drinking.
5. Sip and enjoy the calming and comforting benefits of skullcap, holy basil, and chamomile tea!

Skullcap and Passionflower Tincture

Skullcap and passionflower tincture is an herbal remedy known for its calming effects on the nervous system.

Instructions:

1. Combine equal parts of dried skullcap and passionflower in a clean glass jar.
2. Pour enough alcohol over the herbs to fully cover them, ensuring they are submerged.
3. Seal the jar tightly with a lid and gently mix the ingredients.
4. Place the jar in a cool, dark place for about 4-6 weeks to allow the herbs to infuse into the alcohol, shaking the jar occasionally.
5. After the infusion, strain the liquid through a fine mesh strainer or cheesecloth to remove the herb particles.
6. Transfer the tincture into dark glass bottles with dropper lids for easy use and storage.
7. Take a few drops of the tincture diluted in water or juice to help alleviate stress and promote relaxation.

Traditional Kava Tea

Traditional kava tea is a popular beverage known for its calming and relaxing effects.

Instructions:

1. Measure out the desired amount of kava root powder based on your preference and the serving size.
2. Heat water in a saucepan or kettle until it reaches a gentle boil.

3. Place the kava root powder in a muslin cloth or a strainer bag and immerse it in the hot water.
4. Let the kava root powder steep in the hot water for 10-15 minutes, ensuring it doesn't boil.
5. After steeping, remove the muslin cloth or strainer bag containing the kava root powder from the water.
6. Allow the kava tea to cool down for a few minutes before serving.
7. Pour the kava tea into cups and enjoy its soothing effects. Remember to drink it slowly and savor the taste.

Linden, Chamomile, and Lavender Tea (Can Also Be Used for a Tincture)

Linden, chamomile, and lavender tea is a soothing herbal blend known for its calming properties.

Instructions:

1. Boil water in a kettle or saucepan.
2. Place a teaspoon of dried linden, chamomile, and lavender buds into a teapot or heat-resistant container.
3. Pour the boiling water over the herbs in the teapot.
4. Cover the teapot and let the herbs steep in the hot water for about 5-10 minutes.
5. Strain the tea using a fine mesh strainer or infuser into cups.
6. Optionally, you can sweeten the tea with honey or add a slice of lemon for extra flavor.
7. Enjoy the calming effects of linden, chamomile, and lavender tea as a soothing beverage.

Aloe Vera Juice

Aloe vera juice, known for its health benefits, can be enhanced by adding fruit juice or coconut milk.

Instructions:

1. Begin by carefully extracting the gel from fresh aloe vera leaves. Slice the leaves open lengthwise and scoop out the gel using a spoon.
2. Add the extracted aloe vera gel into a blender.
3. Pour your choice of fruit juice or coconut milk into the blender.
4. Blend the mixture on high speed until smooth and well combined.
5. If using coconut milk, ensure it's well mixed with the aloe vera gel.
6. Transfer the blended mixture into a glass or bottle for storage.
7. Refrigerate the aloe vera juice and consume it chilled for a refreshing and nutritious beverage.
8. Shake or stir well before serving to ensure proper distribution of ingredients.
9. Enjoy the benefits of homemade aloe vera juice with added fruit juice or coconut milk.

Flaxseed and Fennel Crackers

Flaxseed and fennel crackers offer a delightful blend of flavors and health benefits, and they can also be paired together to make a soothing tea.

Instructions:

1. Preheat your oven to the recommended temperature for baking crackers.
2. Combine the ground flaxseeds and finely chopped fennel seeds in a mixing bowl in equal proportions.
3. Add a pinch of salt if desired, although it's optional.
4. Gradually pour water into the mixture, stirring continuously until you achieve a thick, dough-like consistency.
5. Let the mixture sit for a few minutes to allow the flaxseeds to absorb the water and bind the ingredients together.
6. Line a baking sheet with parchment paper or lightly grease it to prevent sticking.
7. Spoon the flaxseed and fennel mixture onto the prepared baking sheet, spreading it evenly with a spatula or spoon.
8. Use a knife or pizza cutter to score the mixture into desired cracker-sized pieces.
9. Place the baking sheet in the oven and bake the crackers until golden brown and crispy, typically for about 15-20 minutes.
10. Once baked, remove the crackers from the oven and let them cool completely before breaking them apart along the scored lines.
11. Store the flaxseed and fennel crackers in an airtight container for freshness.

12. Enjoy these nutritious and flavorful crackers on their own or paired with dips, spreads, or as part of a cheese platter.

Passionflower Vinaigrette

Passionflower vinaigrette offers a unique blend of flavors that pairs well with lemon balm, lavender, and skullcap, creating a delightful addition to salads.

Instructions:

1. Begin by gently washing and drying the passionflower petals or whole flower heads to remove dirt or debris.
2. In a mixing bowl, combine olive oil, apple cider vinegar, Dijon mustard, honey or maple syrup, salt, and pepper in the desired proportions.
3. Whisk the ingredients together until they are well combined and the mixture has a smooth consistency.
4. If using whole flower heads, gently crush them to release their flavors and aromas before adding them to the vinaigrette mixture.
5. Stir the passionflower petals or crushed flower heads into the vinaigrette, ensuring they are evenly distributed throughout the mixture.
6. Taste the vinaigrette and adjust the seasoning or sweetness levels according to your preference.
7. Transfer the passionflower vinaigrette to a clean jar or bottle with a tight-fitting lid for storage.
8. Allow the vinaigrette to sit for at least 30 minutes to allow the flavors to meld together before using it.
9. Shake well before serving and drizzle over your favorite salads, or use it as a marinade for grilled vegetables or proteins.

10. Enjoy the refreshing and floral notes of the passionflower vinaigrette to enhance your culinary creations.

CONCLUSION

The final chapter takes herbal remedies away from the necessary and more toward the nice-to-haves that will still have an incredible impact on well-being and quality of life. It's a bonus about Herbal Remedies for Optimal Well-Being!

BONUS HERBAL REMEDIES FOR OPTIMAL WELL-BEING

In this final chapter, we delve into the diverse applications of medicinal plants beyond chronic illnesses. From addressing hormone balance and menopause to providing safe remedies for children and supporting fertility and pregnancy, herbs offer holistic solutions for various health concerns.

Additionally, we explore how herbal remedies can enhance skincare and promote youthful-looking hair, offering alternative options to conventional treatments and expensive products. Embracing the versatility of herbs empowers readers to optimize their well-being and live life to its fullest potential, naturally and affordably.

EVIDENCE-BASED HERBS FOR CHILDREN

When used in culinary doses, some herbs and spices are generally safe for children, assuming there are no allergic reactions. However, because of their age, there is limited research on the specific effects of herbs on children.

Always exercise caution and consult with a healthcare professional before introducing herbs to children, particularly if they have any underlying health conditions or if they are taking other medications. Always start with small doses and closely monitor for any adverse reactions.

Catnip

Catnip is often used as an evidence-based herbal remedy for children due to its mild sedative properties, which can help alleviate symptoms of restlessness and promote relaxation.

It's commonly administered in small doses, typically as a tea, to help soothe colic, indigestion, or mild anxiety in infants and young children. However, it's essential to consult with a healthcare provider before using catnip or any herbal remedy for children, especially if they have underlying health conditions or if they are taking other medications.

Chamomile

Chamomile is widely recognized as an herbal remedy for children due to its calming and soothing properties. It's often used to ease colic symptoms, teething discomfort, and mild digestive issues in infants and young children.

Chamomile tea is a popular and gentle way to administer this herb to children. Still, parents should consult with a healthcare provider before use, especially if the child has allergies or medical conditions.

Echinacea

Echinacea is an herbal remedy for children, supporting immune function and alleviating symptoms of common colds and respiratory infections. Research suggests that echinacea may help reduce the duration and severity of cold symptoms in children at the onset of illness.

However, parents should exercise caution and consult with a healthcare professional before giving echinacea to children, especially those with autoimmune conditions or allergies.

Licorice

Licorice is recognized as an evidence-based herbal remedy for children due to its potential benefits for soothing coughs and respiratory discomfort. Its demulcent properties make it useful for soothing irritated throats and promoting respiratory health.

However, due to the risk of side effects and interactions, parents must consult healthcare professionals before administering licorice to children, especially in high doses or for extended periods.

Moringa

Moringa is a versatile and evidence-based herbal remedy suitable for children due to its wide range of health benefits. Rich in nutrients and antioxidants, moringa supports overall health, immune function, and growth in children.

Its mild flavor makes it easy to incorporate into various foods and beverages, making it a convenient option for parents looking to naturally enhance their children's nutrition.

MEDICINAL PLANTS FOR FERTILITY

Medicinal plants for fertility offer a natural approach for individuals seeking to enhance their reproductive health. These plants have been traditionally used to support fertility, promoting hormonal balance and reproductive function.

From regulating menstrual cycles to improving sperm health, medicinal plants provide a holistic option for those faced with fertility issues.

Chasteberry

Chasteberry, also known as Vitex agnus-castus, is a popular herb used for enhancing fertility in both men and women. It helps regulate hormonal balance, particularly in irregular menstrual cycles or luteal phase defects.

Chasteberry is believed to support the production of luteinizing hormone (LH), which plays a crucial role in ovulation and menstrual cycle regulation. Many individuals turn to chasteberry as a natural remedy to improve fertility and increase the chances of conception.

Black Cohosh

Black cohosh is often used as an herbal remedy to support fertility and reproductive health, especially in women. It is believed to help regulate menstrual cycles and promote hormonal balance, enhancing fertility.

Additionally, black cohosh is sometimes used to alleviate symptoms of menopause and support overall reproductive wellness. While more research is needed to fully understand its effects on fertility, many women have reported positive outcomes when incorporating black cohosh into their fertility support regimen.

Red Clover

Red clover is commonly used as an herbal remedy to support fertility and reproductive health in women. It contains isoflavones, believed to mimic estrogen in the body and promote hormonal balance.

By helping to regulate the menstrual cycle and support overall reproductive function, red clover may improve fertility outcomes. However, it's essential to consult with a healthcare provider before using red clover or any herbal remedy for fertility to ensure safety and efficacy for individual needs.

Maca

Maca is a renowned herbal remedy to enhance fertility and reproductive health in both men and women. It's believed to support hormonal balance and increase libido, which can improve chances of conception.

Rich in nutrients and adaptogenic compounds, maca has been traditionally used to promote overall vitality and fertility. However, it's advisable to consult with a healthcare professional before using maca or any herbal remedy to address fertility concerns.

Cinnamon

Cinnamon is known for its potential to support fertility by helping regulate menstrual cycles and improve insulin sensitivity. Its anti-inflammatory and antioxidant properties may contribute to reproductive health by reducing oxidative stress.

Including cinnamon into your diet or as a supplement may help promote hormonal balance and support reproductive function, but consulting with a healthcare provider is recommended for personalized advice.

Ashwagandha

Ashwagandha is a revered herb in Ayurvedic medicine, known for its adaptogenic properties that may support fertility by reducing stress levels and balancing hormones. Studies suggest that ashwagandha supplementation could improve sperm quality, ovarian function, and menstrual regularity in both men and women (Cronkleton, 2023).

Its ability to modulate stress hormones like cortisol may also enhance overall reproductive health and increase the chances of conception. However, it's essential to consult with a healthcare professional before incorporating ashwagandha into your fertility regimen.

Dong Quai

Dong quai, also known as "female ginseng," is traditionally used in Chinese medicine to support women's reproductive health and fertility. It is believed to regulate estrogen levels, improve blood circulation to the reproductive organs, and promote a healthy menstrual cycle.

While some women use dong quai to enhance fertility, its safety and effectiveness for this purpose are not well-established, and it's essential to consult with a healthcare provider before using it, especially during pregnancy or while trying to conceive. As with any herbal remedy, individual responses may vary, and caution is advised when considering its use for fertility support.

SUPPORTING A HEALTHY PREGNANCY

Expecting mothers must consult their healthcare providers before using any herbal remedies during pregnancy. While some herbs are considered safe and beneficial for supporting a healthy pregnancy, others can potentially induce uterine contractions and are not recommended.

Discuss herbal supplementation with a healthcare provider to ensure safety and avoid any risks to the mother and baby. Mothers can make informed decisions to support their health and well-being throughout pregnancy by providing guidance on safe herbal options and those to avoid.

Moringa Leaf

Moringa leaf is generally considered safe for consumption during pregnancy and breastfeeding when taken in moderate amounts as part of a balanced diet. It is rich in vitamins, minerals, and antioxidants, which can benefit the mother and the baby.

However, pregnant and breastfeeding women should consult their healthcare providers before incorporating moringa leaf into their diet to ensure it's suitable for their health needs and to avoid potential risks.

Aloe Vera and Gotu Kola

Aloe vera and gotu kola are commonly used in skincare products due to their potential to improve skin health. When combined in a salve, they may help moisturize the skin and improve its elasticity, which could contribute to reducing the appearance of stretch marks over time.

However, individual results may vary, and it's advisable to perform a patch test and consult a dermatologist before applying any new skincare product, especially during pregnancy or breastfeeding.

BALANCING HORMONES THE NATURAL WAY

Balancing hormones naturally can be achieved through various herbs and spices, many of which have multiple health benefits beyond hormone regulation. You can support hormone balance and promote well-being using chasteberry, black cohosh, red clover, and maca.

These versatile botanicals offer holistic solutions that empower you to take charge of your health sustainably and naturally.

Ashwagandha

Ashwagandha, a potent adaptogenic herb, is renowned for supporting hormone balance in the body. By modulating stress levels and reducing cortisol production, ashwagandha helps regulate the endocrine system, promoting hormonal equilibrium.

Its adaptogenic properties make it particularly effective in alleviating symptoms of hormonal imbalance, such as fatigue, mood swings, and irregular menstrual cycles. Using ashwagandha in your daily routine can help restore harmony to your hormonal health, fostering a greater sense of well-being and vitality.

Black Cohosh

Black cohosh is highly valued for its effectiveness in addressing symptoms of menopause, including hot flashes, night sweats, and mood swings. As a natural hormone regulator, black cohosh aids in restoring hormonal balance during this transitional phase in a woman's life.

Its ability to mimic the effects of estrogen in the body helps alleviate discomfort and promote overall well-being, offering women a holistic approach to managing menopausal symptoms.

Maca

Maca, a root vegetable native to Peru, is renowned for its hormone-balancing properties, particularly in women. It acts as an adaptogen, helping the body adapt to stress and supporting the endocrine system's overall function.

Maca is believed to regulate hormone levels, including estrogen and progesterone, which can alleviate symptoms of hormonal imbalance such as irregular menstruation, mood swings, and fatigue.

Chamomile

Chamomile is a gentle yet effective herb that promotes hormone balance, especially in women. It contains compounds that can help regulate menstrual cycles and alleviate symptoms associated with hormonal fluctuations, such as mood swings and irritability.

Additionally, chamomile's calming properties can contribute to emotional well-being during hormonal changes.

Turmeric

Turmeric, a vibrant yellow spice, offers potential benefits for hormone balance. Its active compound, curcumin, exhibits anti-inflammatory properties that may help regulate hormone levels by reducing inflammation.

Studies suggest that turmeric consumption could support hormonal health by promoting a balanced inflammatory response, which is crucial for overall well-being (Gunnars, 2023).

Sage

Sage has aromatic properties but also helps with hormone balance. Its phytoestrogen content helps regulate hormonal fluctuations, particularly in menopausal women experiencing symptoms such as hot flashes and mood swings.

By supporting hormonal equilibrium, sage could contribute to a sense of well-being and improved quality of life during transitional phases such as menopause.

Vitex (Chasteberry)

Vitex, commonly known as chasteberry, is renowned for supporting hormone balance, particularly in women. It works by regulating the production of certain hormones, especially those related to the menstrual cycle.

By promoting hormonal harmony, Vitex may alleviate symptoms of PMS, irregular periods, and other menstrual issues, offering women a natural approach to reproductive health and well-being.

Motherwort

Motherwort, valued for its calming properties, also supports hormone balance, especially in women experiencing menopausal symptoms. Its natural compounds help regulate hormonal fluctuations, easing mood swings and promoting emotional stability.

By including motherwort into their wellness routine, you may find relief from the challenges associated with hormonal changes, fostering a greater sense of balance and tranquility.

Red Clover

Red clover, renowned for its phytoestrogen content, aids in hormone balance, particularly in menopausal women. Its compounds mimic estrogen's effects in the body, alleviating symptoms like hot flashes and mood swings.

Regular consumption of red clover may support hormonal equilibrium, promoting overall well-being during transitional phases in a woman's life.

Yarrow

Yarrow, a versatile herb, assists in hormone balance by regulating menstrual cycles and relieving menstrual discomfort. Its anti-inflammatory and antispasmodic properties may alleviate symptoms such as cramps and bloating.

Additionally, yarrow's astringent qualities support the body's natural hormonal fluctuations, promoting equilibrium.

Dandelion Root

Dandelion root contributes to hormone balance by supporting liver function, which is crucial in metabolizing hormones. Its detoxifying properties help remove excess hormones from the body, promoting balance.

Additionally, dandelion root's ability to reduce inflammation may alleviate symptoms associated with hormonal imbalance.

Red Raspberry Leaf

Red raspberry leaf is often recommended for hormone balance due to its toning effect on the uterus. It is believed to support hormonal health by promoting overall reproductive wellness in women.

Regular red raspberry leaf tea consumption may help regulate menstrual cycles and alleviate symptoms associated with hormonal fluctuations.

RETAINING YOUR YOUTHFUL APPEARANCE

Finally, let's explore how to use herbs for maintaining youthful skin and hair. Many of the herbs and spices previously discussed can also benefit the skin and hair. For instance, rosemary and lavender can be infused into oils for scalp massages, while chamomile and calendula can create soothing skin balms.

Additionally, aloe vera and coconut oil combined with essential oils are useful as hydrating skin treatments or added to baths for a relaxing and nourishing experience. It's all about maximizing what you have to promote natural beauty and well-being.

Chamomile

Chamomile is renowned for its soothing and anti-inflammatory properties, making it a gentle yet effective option for promoting youthful skin. Its antioxidant-rich nature helps combat free radicals, which contribute to premature aging and skin damage.

Adding chamomile to skincare routines, such as using it in facial steams or as a soothing toner, can help maintain a radiant and youthful complexion.

Lavender

Lavender's calming aroma and natural antibacterial properties make it a versatile ingredient for maintaining youthful skin. It can soothe irritation, promote relaxation, and help reduce stress-related aging signs.

Adding a few drops of lavender essential oil to skincare products or using it in DIY face masks can rejuvenate the skin and contribute to a youthful glow.

Stinging Nettle

Stinging nettle, rich in vitamins and minerals, offers numerous benefits for maintaining youthful skin. Its anti-inflammatory properties help soothe irritation and reduce redness, promoting a clearer complexion.

Incorporating nettle extracts or infusions into skincare routines can help combat signs of aging and contribute to a healthier, more radiant appearance.

Peppermint

Peppermint is renowned for its refreshing and invigorating properties, which can rejuvenate tired skin and promote a youthful glow. Its natural menthol content provides a cooling sensation that soothes and revitalizes the skin, leaving it feeling refreshed and renewed.

Using peppermint-infused skincare products or peppermint oil in DIY beauty treatments can help invigorate the skin and maintain a youthful appearance.

Rosemary

Rosemary is celebrated for its antioxidant properties, which can help combat free radicals and protect the skin from premature aging. Its stimulating effect on circulation promotes blood flow to the skin, enhancing its overall tone and vitality.

Rosemary-infused skincare products or rosemary essential oil in massages can revitalize the skin, leaving it radiant and youthful.

Aloe Vera

Aloe vera is renowned for its moisturizing and soothing properties, making it a popular ingredient in skincare products to maintain youthful skin. Rich in vitamins, minerals, and antioxidants, aloe vera helps nourish the skin, keeping it hydrated and supple while reducing the appearance of fine lines and wrinkles.

Regularly applying aloe vera gel or aloe vera products can contribute to a more youthful and radiant complexion.

Turmeric

Turmeric, known for its vibrant yellow color and medicinal properties, offers numerous benefits for maintaining a youthful appearance. Its potent anti-inflammatory and antioxidant properties help protect the skin from damage caused by free radicals, reducing signs of aging such as wrinkles and dark spots.

Adding turmeric to skincare routines through DIY masks or commercial products can promote a clearer, brighter complexion and contribute to overall skin health.

Cinnamon

Cinnamon, celebrated for its warm and spicy aroma, is a kitchen staple and a potent ally in promoting a youthful appearance. Rich in antioxidants, cinnamon helps fight oxidative stress and prevents premature aging by reducing the formation of fine lines and wrinkles.

Whether used in facial masks, scrubs, or consumed in teas, cinnamon invigorates the skin, leaving it refreshed and rejuvenated.

Thyme

With its earthy fragrance and robust flavor, thyme is more than just a culinary herb; it's also a natural aid for maintaining youthful skin. Packed with antioxidants and antibacterial properties, thyme helps combat free radicals and soothes inflammation, promoting a clear complexion.

Whether infused in oils for massages, added to facial steams, or brewed into herbal teas, thyme offers a refreshing boost to the skin, leaving it revitalized and radiant.

Basil

Basil isn't just a flavorful herb for cooking; it also offers numerous benefits for maintaining youthful skin. Rich in antioxidants like vitamin C and other essential nutrients, basil helps protect the skin from environmental damage and premature aging.

Whether used in skincare products, infused into oils for massages, or enjoyed in teas, basil promotes a healthy glow. It can help reduce the appearance of fine lines and wrinkles, leaving your skin refreshed and rejuvenated.

Sage

Sage is renowned for its potent antioxidant properties, making it a valuable ally in skincare routines aimed at maintaining a youthful appearance. Rich in rosmarinic acid and other compounds, sage helps protect the skin from oxidative stress and promotes collagen production, reducing the signs of aging.

Sage in facial steams, herbal baths, or incorporated into skincare formulations can help tighten pores, improve skin texture, and diminish the appearance of fine lines and wrinkles, leaving you with a radiant and youthful complexion.

Dandelion

Dandelion is a powerhouse herb known for its detoxifying and rejuvenating effects on the skin, contributing to a more youthful appearance. Its high content of vitamins A, C, and E, along with minerals such as zinc and selenium, nourishes the skin and promotes collagen production, helping to reduce the appearance of wrinkles and fine lines.

Whether consumed as a tea, incorporated into skincare products, or used as a topical treatment, dandelion can help revitalize the skin, leaving it smoother, brighter, and more youthful.

Explore the versatility of medicinal plants and have fun experimenting with different combinations and applications. By applying this knowledge, you can discover creative ways to harness the power of herbs for health and well-being. With their potent properties, medicinal plants offer endless holistic healing and nourishment possibilities.

Inspire and Empower!

A secure knowledge of herbal healing is a powerful tool in taking charge of your health and quelling your worries... and this is your chance to empower new readers to take this life-changing journey.

Simply by sharing your honest opinion of this book and a little about your own experience, you'll inspire other people to discover the secrets of herbal medicine and enjoy the peace of mind it offers.

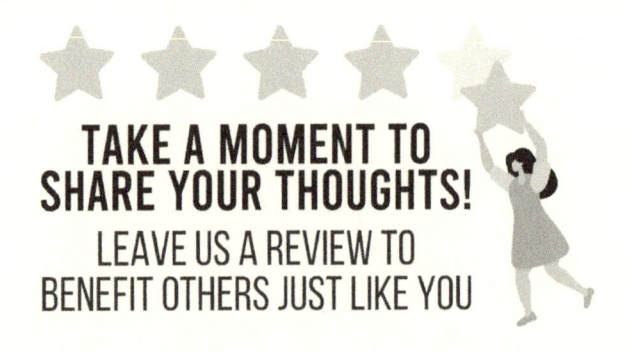

TAKE A MOMENT TO SHARE YOUR THOUGHTS! LEAVE US A REVIEW TO BENEFIT OTHERS JUST LIKE YOU

Thank you so much for your support. It makes a huge difference.

CONCLUSION

Throughout this guide, you've learned the enduring wisdom and efficacy of herbal remedies in maintaining holistic health and wellness. The central message resonates throughout its pages: nature offers abundant resources for healing and restoration.

Stress, lifestyle choices, and environmental factors profoundly influence our health, often challenging the delicate balance within our bodies. Herbal remedies are your allies, offering gentle yet potent solutions to address imbalances and promote vitality.

By harnessing the power of herbal remedies, you can mitigate the effects of stress, adapt to changing lifestyles, and counteract environmental stressors. Herbal remedies offer a natural, sustainable approach to health maintenance, rooted in centuries of traditional knowledge and modern scientific validation.

As we end our wellness journey, let us embrace the simplicity and potency of herbal remedies, nurturing our bodies, minds, and spirits in harmony with the wisdom of nature.

KEY TAKEAWAYS

- **Harness Nature's Bounty**: We emphasized the abundant healing potential found in nature's botanical treasures. From calming chamomile to immune-boosting echinacea, herbal remedies offer diverse solutions for various health concerns.
- **Start Holistic Healing**: Herbal remedies highlight the importance of holistic health, addressing physical symptoms and mental and emotional well-being. By treating the whole person, these remedies foster balance and vitality from within.
- **Learn Timeless Wisdom** and **Modern Validation**: While rooted in ancient traditions, herbal remedies find validation in contemporary scientific research. Their effectiveness in combating stress, supporting immune function, and enhancing overall health is increasingly recognized and studied.
- **Consider Lifestyle Integration**: Incorporating herbal remedies into daily life promotes a proactive approach to health maintenance. You can cultivate resilience and vitality by making conscious choices about nutrition, self-care practices, and environmental factors.
- **Learn Great Knowledge**: You now understand herbal remedies and their potential benefits. You can take proactive steps toward self-care and naturally optimize your health and well-being.

THE BEST HERBS FOR OVERALL WELLNESS

Which are your favorite herbs so far? Here are the most versatile and potent herbs, flowers, and plants. Be sure to include these in your cooking and daily wellness routines.

Basil (Ocimum basilicum)

- Basil possesses anti-inflammatory and antioxidant properties. It also aids digestion and supports cardiovascular health.
- Use fresh basil in salads, sandwiches, and pasta dishes or as a garnish for soups. It can also be brewed into tea or incorporated into herbal remedies for digestive issues.

Rosemary (Rosmarinus officinalis)

- Rosemary is rich in antioxidants and anti-inflammatory compounds. It may improve memory and concentration, support digestion, and have antimicrobial properties.
- Add fresh or dried rosemary to roasted vegetables, meats, soups, and bread for flavor. Rosemary-infused oil can also be used for massage or aromatherapy.

Mint (Mentha spp.)

- Mint is known for its calming effect on the digestive system, relieving indigestion, nausea, and gas. It also has antimicrobial properties and can freshen breath.
- Use fresh mint leaves in salads, smoothies, teas, and desserts. Mint oil can be applied topically for headache relief or used in aromatherapy.

Turmeric (Curcuma longa)

- Turmeric contains curcumin, a compound with potent anti-inflammatory and antioxidant properties. It may help alleviate joint pain, reduce inflammation, and support cognitive function.
- Add turmeric powder to curries, soups, smoothies, and stir-fries for a vibrant color and earthy flavor. Turmeric tea and golden milk are popular ways to consume it for health benefits.

Ginger (Zingiber officinale)

- Ginger is well-known for its anti-nausea properties and can help alleviate motion and morning sickness. It also has anti-inflammatory and antioxidant effects, supporting digestive health and reducing muscle pain.
- Use fresh ginger in teas, stir-fries, marinades, and soups. Ginger supplements or ginger chews are also available for digestive support.

Garlic (Allium sativum)

- Garlic contains allicin, a compound with potent antimicrobial and immune-boosting properties. It may help lower blood pressure and cholesterol levels and reduce the risk of cardiovascular disease.
- Add minced or crushed garlic to sauces, dressings, marinades, and roasted vegetables for flavor and health benefits. Raw garlic can also be consumed for its immune-boosting effects.

Lavender (Lavandula angustifolia)

- Lavender has calming and stress-relieving properties, promoting relaxation and sleep. It may also help alleviate anxiety, headaches, and mild pain.
- For aromatherapy and relaxation, use dried lavender flowers to make teas, sachets, bath salts, and infused oils. Lavender essential oil can be diluted and applied topically for skin irritation or used in diffusers for aromatherapy.

Chamomile (Matricaria chamomilla)

- Chamomile is renowned for its calming and soothing effects on the nervous system, promoting relaxation and improving sleep quality. It also has anti-inflammatory and digestive properties.
- Brew chamomile flowers into tea for a calming bedtime ritual. Chamomile tea can also be used topically as a rinse for skin irritation or inflammation.

Cinnamon (Cinnamomum verum)

- Cinnamon contains powerful antioxidants and has anti-inflammatory properties. It may help regulate blood sugar levels, improve heart health, and boost cognitive function.
- Add cinnamon powder to oatmeal, smoothies, baked goods, and savory dishes for warmth and flavor. Cinnamon sticks can infuse flavor into teas, mulled wine, and desserts.

Echinacea (Echinacea purpurea)

- Echinacea is widely used to support the immune system and reduce the severity and duration of colds and the flu. It also has anti-inflammatory and antioxidant properties.
- Brew echinacea roots or flowers into teas, tinctures, or extracts to support immune function during cold and flu season. Echinacea supplements are also available in various forms for immune support.

These herbs, spices, and flowers offer many health benefits and can be easily incorporated into daily meals, teas, and remedies to support overall well-being.

YOU'RE INVITED TO A WELLNESS JOURNEY!

The road to a beautiful, healthy, new you begins today! The journey does not have to be daunting or complicated, and it starts right in your kitchen with the herbs and spices you already have on hand. By exploring the healing potential within your spice rack, you can initiate a transformative journey toward holistic health and well-being.

This book is not just about herbs and remedies; it's about reclaiming control over health, nurturing your body with nature's gifts, and fostering a deeper connection to the natural world.

May you find abundance, vitality, and joy in embracing herbal remedies and holistic living.

Your review matters! Please take time to review this guide. Your message and experience using herbal remedies can help others struggling with health concerns or fears. By sharing your practical and effective solutions, you can inspire and empower others to take charge of their health and embrace natural remedies.

REFERENCES

10 home remedies to naturally reduce stretch marks | Mederma®. (2023, July 5). mederma.com. https://www.mederma.com/article/10-home-remedies-to-naturally-reduce-stretch-marks/

21 Best Herbs and spices for skin care: Benefits and how to use them. (2023, December 15). STYLECRAZE. https://www.stylecraze.com/articles/best-herbs-and-spices-for-skin/

ADI - Dementia statistics. (n.d.). ADI - Dementia Statistics. https://www.alzint.org/about/dementia-facts-figures/dementia-statistics/

Admin. (n.d.). *Licorice and respiratory health.* https://albertparknaturopathy.com.au/licorice-and-respiratory-health/

Aishwarya, A., & Aishwarya, A. (2023, December 19). *How to use saffron in milk for fairness?* Foodnutra - Online Shop Flavoured Dry Fruits and Premium Spices. https://www.foodnutra.com/how-to-use-saffron-in-milk-for-fairness/

Alieta. (n.d.). *How to make a cooling herbal compress in 3 easy steps.* https://blog.mountainroseherbs.com/cooling-herbal-compress-3-easy-steps

Aloe vera for your bowels | Constipation, IBS, gut health | H&B. (2023, August 21). https://www.hollandandbarrett.com/the-health-hub/conditions/digestive-health/is-aloe-vera-good-for-your-bowels/#

Alphafoodie. (2022, April 19). *How to make aloe vera juice.* https://www.alphafoodie.com/how-to-make-aloe-vera-juice/

Alphafoodie. (2024, February 21). *DIY turmeric tincture – Nature's golden medicine.* https://www.alphafoodie.com/turmeric-tincture-natures-golden-medicine/

American Lung Association. (n.d.). *Our impact.* https://www.lung.org/about-us/our-impact

American Pregnancy Association. (2022, June 9). *Herbs and pregnancy.* https://americanpregnancy.org/healthy-pregnancy/is-it-safe/herbs-and-pregnancy/

Anonymous. (2021a, March 18). *The Anti-Inflammatory potential of rosemary.* Designs for Health. https://www.casi.org/node/1378

Anonymous. (2021b, September 2). *The relaxing effects of chamomile.* Designs for Health. https://www.casi.org/node/1451

Atkins Expert Sinus Care. (2023, November 2). *Peppermint oil to treat allergies.* AESC. https://www.atkinssinus.com/peppermint-oil-to-treat-allergies/#:

Babar, F. (2023, July 26). *Taking moringa during and after pregnancy.* Moringa Vinga.

https://moringavinga.com/blogs/health-wellness/taking-moringa-during-and-after-pregnancy

Bcps, R. P. P. B. B. (2023, October 5). What are the benefits of Devil's Claw? *Verywell Health*. https://www.verywellhealth.com/devils-claw-what-should-i-know-about-it-89445

Bhattacharya, V., Mishra, N., Sharma, R. R., Dubey, S. K., Chandrasekaran, B., & Bayan, M. F. (2023). Recent targeted discovery of phytomedicines to manage endocrine disorder develops due to adapting sedentary lifestyle. In *Elsevier eBooks* (pp. 143–161). https://doi.org/10.1016/b978-0-443-19143-5.00021-9

Black pepper health benefits. (n.d.). HerbalRemediesAdvice.org. https://www.herbalremediesadvice.org/black-pepper-health-benefits.html

Blau, K. (2023, August 18). *Goldenrod benefits: the bee's knees for allergies, sinus infections, and urinary tract infections*. Chestnut School of Herbal Medicine. https://chestnutherbs.com/goldenrod-flower/

Boushee, M. (2023, October 16). *How to use saffron & Make saffron milk*. LearningHerbs. https://learningherbs.com/remedies-recipes/how-to-use-saffron/

Bramlet, K. (2019, August 6). Phytochemicals and cancer: What you should know. *MD Anderson Cancer Center*. https://www.mdanderson.org/publications/focused-on-health/phytochemicals-and-cancer-what-you-should-know.h10-1591413.html#:

BSc, K. G. (2023, November 27). *10 Health benefits of tumeric and curcumin*. Healthline. https://www.healthline.com/nutrition/top-10-evidence-based-health-benefits-of-turmeric

Bsn, S. a. W. R. (2021, December 16). *All About Kava: Can It Help with Anxiety and Mental Health?* Psych Central. https://psychcentral.com/anxiety/what-is-kava#what-it-is

Cafasso, J. (2023, August 31). *Steam inhalation: What are the benefits?* Healthline. https://www.healthline.com/health/steam-inhalation#_noHeaderPrefixedContent

Calming and anti-anxiety benefits of Passionflower — Culinary Witch. (n.d.). Culinary Witch. https://culinarywitch.com/calming-and-antianxiety-benefits-of-passionflower#:

Castro, J. (2014, March 14). *GASP! 11 Surprising Facts about the respiratory System*. livescience.com. https://www.livescience.com/44105-respiratory-system-surprising-facts.html

Chen, B. H., Hsieh, C., Tsai, S. Y., Wang, C. Y., & Wang, C. C. (2020). Anticancer effects of epigallocatechin-3-gallate nanoemulsion on lung cancer cells through the activation of AMP-activated protein kinase signaling pathway. *Scientific Reports*, *10*(1). https://doi.org/10.1038/s41598-020-62136-2

Chen, Y., Lin, L., Wu, L., Xu, Y., Shergis, J. L., Zhang, A. L., Wen, Z., Worsnop, C., Da Costa, C., Thien, F., & Xue, C. C. (2020). <p>Effect of Panax Ginseng (G115) Capsules versus Placebo on Acute Exacerbations in Patients with Moderate to Very Severe COPD: A Randomized Controlled Trial</p> *International Journal of Chronic Obstructive Pulmonary Disease, Volume 15*, 671–680. https://doi.org/10.2147/copd.s236425

Chung, B. (n.d.). *2 Easy ways to use hawthorn berries | Nature with Us*. naturewithus.com. https://naturewithus.com/articles/medicinal-plants/2-easy-ways-to-use-hawthorn-berries

Ciongoli, C. (2021, November 19). *How infused oils are made and how they can transform your cooking - Salute Santé! Grapeseed oil*. Salute Santé! Grapeseed Oil. https://grapeseedoil.com/how-infused-oils-are-made-and-how-they-can-transform-your-cooking/#:

Clinic, C. (2023, December 5). *Is elderberry really an effective cold and flu cure?* Cleveland Clinic. https://health.clevelandclinic.org/is-elderberry-really-an-effective-cold-and-flu-cure

Clinic, C. (2024, January 12). *How Mullein benefits your lungs*. Cleveland Clinic. https://health.clevelandclinic.org/mullein-benefits

Common Myths about Herbal Medicine – Bloom Institute. (n.d.). https://bloominstitute.ca/common-myths-about-herbal-medicine/

Common-Cold tea. (2019, January 22). Martha Stewart. https://www.marthastewart.com/1155943/common-cold-tea

Concio, C. J. H. (2024, January 22). *Thyme can reduce blood pressure and lower the risk of heart disease*. Science Times. https://www.sciencetimes.com/articles/22962/20190624/thyme-can-reduce-blood-pressure-and-lower-the-risk-of-heart-disease.htm

Cronkleton, E. (2023, September 21). *Does ashwagandha make you fertile? 7 things to know About this herb*. Healthline. https://www.healthline.com/health/does-ashwagandha-make-you-fertile

Davinelli, S., Maes, M., Corbi, G., Zarrelli, A., Willcox, D. C., & Scapagnini, G. (2016). Dietary phytochemicals and neuro-inflammaging: from mechanistic insights to translational challenges. *Immunity & Ageing, 13*(1). https://doi.org/10.1186/s12979-016-0070-3

Dementia prevention: Reduce your risk, starting now. (2022, October 12). Johns Hopkins Medicine. https://www.hopkinsmedicine.org/health/conditions-and-diseases/dementia/dementia-prevention-reduce-your-risk

Does eating ginger increase blood pressure? (n.d.). Vinmec. https://www.vinmec.com/en/news/health-news/nutrition/does-eating-ginger-increase-blood-pressure/#:

El-Saadony, M. T., Yang, T., Korma, S. A., Sitohy, M., El–Mageed, T. a. A., Selim,

176 | REFERENCES

S., Jaouni, S. K. A., Salem, H. M., Mahmmod, Y., Soliman, S. M., Momen, S., Mosa, W. F. A., El-Wafai, N. A., Abou-Aly, H. E., Sitohy, B., El-Hack, M. E. A., El-Tarabily, K. A., & Saad, A. M. (2023). Impacts of turmeric and its principal bioactive curcumin on human health: Pharmaceutical, medicinal, and food applications: A comprehensive review. *Frontiers in Nutrition, 9.* https://doi.org/10.3389/fnut.2022.1040259

Eske, J. (2019, April 3). *How does oxidative stress affect the body?* https://www.medicalnewstoday.com/articles/324863#what-is-it

Esmaeili, F., Zahmatkeshan, M., Yousefpoor, Y., Alipanah, H., Safari, E., & Osanloo, M. (2022). Anti-inflammatory and anti-nociceptive effects of Cinnamon and Clove essential oils nanogels: an in vivo study. *BMC Complementary Medicine and Therapies, 22*(1). https://doi.org/10.1186/s12906-022-03619-9

Farm, J. (2024, January 4). *How to make the most effective Hawthorn berry syrup heart tonic.* Joybilee® Farm | DIY | Herbs | Gardening |. https://joybileefarm.com/hawthorn-syrup-heart-tonic/

Fisher, M. Z., & Fisher, M. Z. (2022, May 26). Steam inhalation: How to use fresh herbs to make your own home remedy for congestion relief. *Business Insider.* https://www.businessinsider.com/guides/health/treatments/best-herbs-for-steam-inhalation

Francis, B., & Francis, B. (2021, September 13). *Benefits of Nettle: How to reduce inflammation in the body fast.* The Wild Nettle Co. https://thewildnettleco.com/how-to-reduce-inflammation-in-the-body-fast-with-nettles/

Ghasemian, M., Owlia, S., & Owlia, M. B. (2016). Review of Anti-Inflammatory Herbal Medicines. *Advances in Pharmacological Sciences, 2016,* 1–11. https://doi.org/10.1155/2016/9130979

Gilmore, M. (2021, September 22). *Easy cinnamon tea.* Detoxinista. https://detoxinista.com/cinnamon-tea/

Gis. (2021, July 6). *Peppermint and IBS Pain Relief - Gastrointestinal Society.* Gastrointestinal Society. https://badgut.org/information-centre/a-z-digestive-topics/peppermint-and-ibs-pain-relief/

Gluck, S. (2019, November 6). *De-stress with lemon balm - Marion Gluck.* Marion Gluck. https://www.mariongluckclinic.com/blog/chilling-out-with-lemon-balm.html

Grieve, K. (2021, November 2). *Homemade Hawthorn Berry Ketchup.* Larder Love. https://larderlove.com/hawthorn-ketchup/

Healthdirect Australia. (n.d.). *Circulatory system.* Healthdirect. https://www.healthdirect.gov.au/circulatory-system#:

Heidi. (n.d.). *8 Best herbs for natural skin care.* https://blog.mountainroseherbs.com/8-of-the-best-herbs-for-natural-skin-care

REFERENCES | 177

Heidi. (2019, January 3). *Soothing wild cherry bark syrup recipe for a dry throat.* https://blog.mountainroseherbs.com/soothing-throat-syrup

Helmenstine, A. M., PhD. (2020, February 3). *List of medicines made from plants.* ThoughtCo. https://www.thoughtco.com/drugs-and-medicine-made-from-plants-608413

Herbal Clinic - Swansea. (2018, August 10). *Brief History Herbal Medicine - Herbal Clinic - Swansea.* https://www.herbalclinic-swansea.co.uk/herbal-medicine/a-brief-history-of-herbal-medicine/

Herbal History. (2021, February 1). Herbal Academy. https://theherbalacademy.com/herbal-history/

Herbal Medicine. (2021, September 24). Johns Hopkins Medicine. https://www.hopkinsmedicine.org/health/wellness-and-prevention/herbal-medicine

Herbal Reality. (2023, December 4). *Licorice - Herbal Reality.* https://www.herbalreality.com/herb/licorice/

Herbal salves. (n.d.). Quiet Creek Herb Farm & School of Country Living. https://www.quietcreekherbfarm.org/herbal-salves.html#:

Herbaugh, T. M. (2021, September 6). *Borage seed oil for rheumatoid arthritis.* https://www.medicalnewstoday.com/articles/borage-seed-oil-rheumatoid-arthritis#borage-seed-oil

Herbs for kids: What's safe, what's not. (2000, June 25). WebMD. https://www.webmd.com/balance/features/herbs-for-kids-feature

Herbs, I. (2020). Wild cherry benefits. *Indigo Herbs.* https://www.indigo-herbs.co.uk/natural-health-guide/benefits/wild-cherry

How to feed children moringa? (n.d.). Vinmec. https://www.vinmec.com/en/news/health-news/nutrition/how-to-feed-children-moringa/

How to make ashwagandha tincture. (2023, February 27). LA Herb. https://laherb.com/blogs/tincture-recipes/how-to-make-ashwagandha-tincture#:

How to make herbal teas and infusions — Community Pharmacy. (2022, April 7). Community Pharmacy. https://www.communitypharmacy.coop/blog/how-to-make-herbal-teas-and-infusions#:

How your brain makes and uses energy. (2024, February 7). Queensland Brain Institute - University of Queensland. https://qbi.uq.edu.au/brain/nature-discovery/how-your-brain-makes-and-uses-energy

Iftikhar, N., MD. (2019, July 23). *Fennel seeds for fighting gas.* Healthline. https://www.healthline.com/health/fennel-seeds-for-gas

Inflammation and your health. (n.d.). https://www.cedars-sinai.org/discoveries/inflammation.html

J, K. (2021, June 25). *ORAC Value List – Top 100 Highest Antioxidant Spices, Herbs, products.* Modern Survival Blog. https://modernsurvivalblog.com/health/high-orac-value-antioxidant-foods-top-100/

178 | REFERENCES

Jack. (2023, April 6). *5 herbs to supercharge your immune system*. College of Naturopathic Medicine. https://www.naturopathy-uk.com/news/blog/2023/04/05/5-herbs-to-supercharge-your-immune-system/

Jacob, L. (2023, November 8). *The best herbal teas for lung health - NutraTea*. NutraTea. https://nutratea.co.uk/herbal-teas-lung-health/

Jill. (2023, December 14). *Medicinal herb gardening for beginners*. The Beginner's Garden. https://journeywithjill.net/gardening/2019/09/10/medicinal-herb-gardening-for-beginners/

Juma, N. (2023, December 10). *130 quotes on stress and how to handle it*. Everyday Power. https://everydaypower.com/stress-quotes/

Justis, A. (2021, August 27). *How to make an herbal syrup – Herbal Academy*. Herbal Academy. https://theherbalacademy.com/herbal-syrup/

Kearney, G. (2024, January 8). *Herbal Medicine Blog — Herbs & Owls*. Herbs & Owls. https://herbsandowls.com/herbal-medicine-blog/brain-boosters-herbs-for-cognitive-support#:

Kenneally, C. (2021, October 21). *Cayenne pepper: the anti-inflammatory and heart healthy spice*. Mediterranean Living. https://www.mediterraneanliving.com/heat-things-up-for-a-healthy-heart/

Kluge, L. (2018, October 30). *March Steep | Chamomile, Linden, Motherwort, Lavender & Peppermint | Ginger Tonic Botanicals*. Ginger Tonic Botanicals. https://www.gingertonicbotanicals.com/blog/march-steep-chamomile-linden-motherwort-lavender-peppermint/

Krans, B. (2020, November 3). *The health benefits of Holy basil*. Healthline. https://www.healthline.com/health/food-nutrition/basil-benefits#:

Kurapati, K. R. V., Atluri, V. S. R., Samikkannu, T., & Nair, M. (2013). Ashwagandha (Withania somnifera) Reverses β-Amyloid1-42 Induced Toxicity in Human Neuronal Cells: Implications in HIV-Associated Neurocognitive Disorders (HAND). *PLOS ONE, 8*(10), e77624. https://doi.org/10.1371/journal.pone.0077624

Ld, L. S. M. R. (2018, August 8). *10 health benefits of cardamom, backed by science*. Healthline. https://www.healthline.com/nutrition/cardamom-benefits#TOC_TITLE_HDR_4

Ld, L. W. M. R. (2023, July 24). *8 Surprising benefits of Linden Tea*. Healthline. https://www.healthline.com/nutrition/linden-tea

Leech, J. (2019, May 27). *The Gut-Brain axis explained in plain English*. https://www.linkedin.com/pulse/gut-brain-axis-explained-plain-english-joe-johan-leech/

Limited, M. (2024, January 18). *What can I put in my diffuser besides oil?* MOZZIN Limited. https://www.mozzinaroma.com/what-can-i-put-in-my-diffuser-besides-oil.html#:

Lomas, K. (n.d.). *Does concentrated thought burn calories?* BBC Science Focus

Magazine. https://www.sciencefocus.com/the-human-body/does-concentrated-thought-burn-calories

Macfarlane, S. (2023, October 18). *9 herbs you need to try for hormone balance.* Wild Dispensary. https://wilddispensary.co.nz/blogs/news/herbs-for-hormone-balance

Make Korean ginseng tea and boost your vitality with this recipe. (2023, February 8). The Spruce Eats. https://www.thespruceeats.com/homemade-korean-ginseng-tea-insam-cha-recipe-2118533

McGruther, J. (2019, July 10). *Nettle infusion.* Nourished Kitchen. https://nourishedkitchen.com/stinging-nettle-infusion/#:

Medicinal botany - plant parts used. (n.d.). https://www.fs.usda.gov/wildflowers/ethnobotany/medicinal/parts.shtml

Meyer, A. (2023, September 17). What happens to your body when you eat reishi mushrooms. *EatingWell.* https://www.eatingwell.com/article/8069689/health-benefits-of-reishi-mushrooms/#:

Mh. (2023, December 21). Busting the common myths about herbal medicine - College of Medicine and Healing Arts. *College of Medicine and Healing Arts.* https://comha.org.uk/busting-the-common-myths-about-herbal-medicine/

Miller, R. (2023, November 6). *Starting a medicinal garden — Zhi Herbals.* Zhi Herbals. https://www.zhiherbals.com/blog/guide-to-starting-a-medicinal-herb-garden

Nordqvist, J. (2023, November 13). *The health benefits of eucalyptus.* https://www.medicalnewstoday.com/articles/266580#benefits-and-uses

North, D. (2023, July 26). *Lion's Mane for Focus: Does it work?* Mission C. https://www.missionc.com/blogs/news/lion-s-mane-for-focus-does-it-work

O'Connor, V. (2022, August 14). Sustainable living: This rosemary tincture recipe can help lift your lethargy and battle brain fog. *Independent.ie.* https://www.independent.ie/life/health-wellbeing/sustainable-living-this-rosemary-tincture-recipe-can-help-lift-your-lethargy-and-battle-brain-fog/41901215.html#:

Office of Dietary Supplements - Ashwagandha: Is it helpful for stress, anxiety, or sleep? (n.d.). https://ods.od.nih.gov/factsheets/Ashwagandha-HealthProfessional/#:

Pakzad, R. (2023, January 10). *8 herbs for hormone balance.* Feminade. https://feminade.com/blogs/nutrition-supplements/herbs-for-hormone-balance

Parmar, R. (2024, February 20). *11 Incredible health benefits of coconut water.* PharmEasy Blog. https://pharmeasy.in/blog/11-incredible-health-benefits-of-coconut-water/#:

Passionflower. (n.d.-a). Mount Sinai Health System. https://www.mountsinai.org/health-library/herb/passionflower#:

Passionflower. (n.d.-b). Flowerfolk Herbal Apothecary | Herbalist Steph Zabel |

Boston, MA. http://www.flowerfolkherbs.com/articles/passionflower#:

Personal stories - Dementia UK. (n.d.). Dementia UK. https://www.dementiauk.org/information-and-support/stories/

Pfeiffer, T. (2021, November 2). This womans journey of recovery from chronic inflammation will inspire you today. *Prevention.* https://www.prevention.com/health/a20498158/chronic-inflammation/

Pgdcr, N. M. B. (2022, September 8). *11 Surprising benefits of parsley tea and how to make it.* MedicineNet. https://www.medicinenet.com/surprising_benefits_of_parsley_tea/article.htm

Pole, S. (2023, August 7). *How to make a decoction.* Earthsong Seeds. https://earthsongseeds.co.uk/recipes/how-to-make-a-decoction/

Professional, C. C. M. (n.d.-a). *inflammation.* Cleveland Clinic. https://my.clevelandclinic.org/health/symptoms/21660-inflammation

Professional, C. C. M. (n.d.-b). *Pneumonitis.* Cleveland Clinic. https://my.clevelandclinic.org/health/diseases/24810-pneumonitis

Puristry. (n.d.). *6 cooking oils you can use on your skin.* Puristry. https://www.puristry.com/blogs/the-routine/6-cooking-oils-you-can-use-on-your-skin

Rapaport, L. (2023, September 22). Ginger may reduce inflammation in autoimmune diseases. *EverydayHealth.com.* https://www.everydayhealth.com/autoimmune-diseases/ginger-may-help-reduce-inflammation-in-autoimmune-diseases/

Raychel. (2017, September 17). *How to make herbal tinctures.* https://blog.mountainroseherbs.com/guide-tinctures-extracts

Rd, A. D. (2022, January 17). *How to make homemade dried herb mix.* Craving Something Healthy. https://cravingsomethinghealthy.com/how-to-make-your-own-dried-herb-mix/

Rd, R. a. M. (2019, December 6). *Can echinacea help you fight the common cold?* Healthline. https://www.healthline.com/nutrition/echinacea-for-colds#:

Rdn, R. C. W. M. (2023, February 20). *What is celery seed?* Verywell Health. https://www.verywellhealth.com/the-benefits-of-celery-seed-88621

Richard Whelan ~ Medical Herbalist ~ Skullcap. (n.d.). https://www.rjwhelan.co.nz/herbs%20A-Z/skullcap.html

Ruscio. (2024, January 17). Oil of Oregano Benefits: How it can Help your health. *Dr. Michael Ruscio, DC.* https://drruscio.com/oil-of-oregano-benefits/

Ruth, T. (2023, October 16). *How to make herbal salves.* LearningHerbs. https://learningherbs.com/remedies-recipes/how-to-make-herbal-salves/

S, J. (2018, March 7). *Holy basil – a key herb for stress, anxiety, depression and fatigue.* https://www.linkedin.com/pulse/20140915021532-5316613-holy-basil-a-key-herb-for-stress-anxiety-depression-and-fatigue/

Sagorchev, P., Lukanov, J., & Am, B. (2010). Investigations into the specific effects of rosemary oil at the receptor level. *Phytomedicine, 17*(8–9), 693–697. https://doi.org/10.1016/j.phymed.2009.09.012

Sawmill Herb Farm. (n.d.). *Herb Profile: Skullcap.* https://www.sawmillherbfarm.com/pages/herb-profile-skullcap#:

Schneider, A. (2020, March 2). *Moringa Tea {a simple and frugal healing tea}.* Creative Simple Living. https://www.schneiderpeeps.com/healing-moringa-tea/#:

Shauli, N. (2022, December 9). *Herbs for fertility.* ELITE IVF - Global IVF Clinic. https://www.elite-ivf.com/herbs-for-fertility/

Shin, J., Ryu, J. H., Kang, M. J., Hwang, C. J., Han, J., & Kang, D. (2013). Short-term heating reduces the anti-inflammatory effects of fresh raw garlic extracts on the LPS-induced production of NO and pro-inflammatory cytokines by down-regulating allicin activity in RAW 264.7 macrophages. *Food and Chemical Toxicology, 58,* 545–551. https://doi.org/10.1016/j.fct.2013.04.002

Simple Kava drink recipe: How to make traditional kava tea - Australian Kava Co. (2022, April 29). *Australian Kava Co.* https://australiankava.com.au/traditional-kava-drink-recipe/

Sonali Ruder, Health & Wellness Writer. (2023, June 9). *Does Mint help you focus?* Life Extension. https://www.lifeextension.com/wellness/herbs-spices/does-mint-help-you-focus

Stephen. (n.d.). *Fragro Plants - Catnip tea.* https://fragroplants.com/index.php/recipes/271-catnip-tea

Stinging nettle. (n.d.). Mount Sinai Health System. https://www.mountsinai.org/health-library/herb/stinging-nettle#:

Stinson, A. (2023, July 26). *Benefits of passionflower for anxiety and insomnia.* https://www.medicalnewstoday.com/articles/323795#what-is-passionflower

Stobart, A. (2024, February 25). *Making herbal poultices and compresses.* Medicinal Forest Garden Trust. https://medicinalforestgardentrust.org/making-herbal-poultices-and-compresses/

Stress and the digestive system. (n.d.). Counseling and Psychological Services (CAPS). https://caps.byu.edu/stress-and-the-digestive-system

Stress symptoms: Effects on your body and behavior. (2023, August 10). Mayo Clinic. https://www.mayoclinic.org/healthy-lifestyle/stress-management/in-depth/stress-symptoms/art-20050987

Sullivan, W. (2014, September 29). *India's Holy Basil - Fresh Cup Magazine.* Fresh Cup Magazine. https://freshcup.com/holy-basil/#:

Summer, J., & Summer, J. (2023, December 20). *Valerian root for sleep.* Sleep Foundation. https://www.sleepfoundation.org/sleep-aids/valerian-root

The Lancet: One in three cases of dementia could be prevented by. (2020, February 13). Psychiatry. https://medicine.umich.edu/dept/psychiatry/news/archive/

182 | REFERENCES

201707/lancet-one-three-cases-dementia-could-be-prevented-targeting-risk-factors-childhood-onwards

The Royal Women's Hospital. (n.d.). *Complementary medicines and breastfeeding.* https://www.thewomens.org.au/health-information/breastfeeding/medicines-drugs-and-breastfeeding/complementary-medicines-and-breastfeeding

The smell of lavender is relaxing, science confirms. (2018, October 18). ScienceDaily. https://www.sciencedaily.com/releases/2018/10/181023085648.htm

tonika health. (2023, March 14). *Myths on Natural Therapies Busted. Read on to learn more..* Acupuncture | Massage | Herbal Med. https://tonikahealth.com.au/7-myths-on-natural-therapies-busted/

TOP 25 HEART DISEASE QUOTES (of 110) | A-Z Quotes. (n.d.). A-Z Quotes. https://www.azquotes.com/quotes/topics/heart-disease.html

TOP 25 HERBS QUOTES (of 204). A-Z Quotes. Accessed March 26, 2024. https://www.azquotes.com/quotes/topics/herbs.html

Uk, B. &. B., Uk, B. &. B., & Uk, B. &. B. (2023, June 27). *What do we know about flaxseed and bowel health?* Bladder & Bowel UK -. https://www.bbuk.org.uk/flaxseed-and-bowel-health/

Upraising. (n.d.). *Flow State - Functional coffee boosted with Lion's Mane, Bacopa Monieri, L-Theanine | Upraising.* https://upraising.co/products/flow-state-coffee-lionsmane-bacopa-ltheanine

Van Den Berg, J. (2018, August 8). All about growing saffron from Crocus sativus bulbs. *Farmer Gracy.* https://www.farmergracy.co.uk/blogs/farmer-gracys-blog/growing-saffron-from-crocus-sativus-bulbs#:

Vicky, K. &. (2022, June 30). *Recipe: Nettle seed joint balm — Handmade Apothecary.* Handmade Apothecary. https://www.handmadeapothecary.co.uk/blog/2021/5/3/nettle-seed-joint-balm

WebMD Editorial Contributor. (2020a, August 24). *Health benefits of basil.* WebMD. https://www.webmd.com/diet/health-benefits-basil

WebMD Editorial Contributor. (2020b, November 12). *Health benefits of Gotu Kola.* WebMD. https://www.webmd.com/diet/health-benefits-gotu-kola

WebMD Editorial Contributors. (2020, December 3). *Catnip tea: Are there health benefits?* WebMD. https://www.webmd.com/diet/catnip-tea-health-benefits

Website, N. (2022, October 19). *Herbal medicines.* nhs.uk. https://www.nhs.uk/conditions/herbal-medicines/#:

What are adaptogens and should you be taking them? (2022, February 16). UCLA Health. https://www.uclahealth.org/news/what-are-adaptogens-and-should-you-be-taking-them#:

What are phytochemicals? (And why should you eat more of them?). (2023, May 10). UCLA Health. https://www.uclahealth.org/news/what-are-phytochemicals-and-why-should-you-eat-more-them

Whole-wheat flaxseed and fennel crackers. (n.d.). Spoonacular. https://spoonacular.com/recipes/whole-wheat-flaxseed-and-fennel-crackers-665301

Wikipedia contributors. (2024, February 22). *History of herbalism.* Wikipedia. https://en.wikipedia.org/wiki/History_of_herbalism

World Health Organization: WHO. (2023, August 10). *Traditional medicine has a long history of contributing to conventional medicine and continues to hold promise.* https://www.who.int/news-room/feature-stories/detail/traditional-medicine-has-a-long-history-of-contributing-to-conventional-medicine-and-continues-to-hold-promise

Yamada, H. (2022). Benefits of green tea: Clinical evidence for respiratory tract infections. *Journal of the Pharmaceutical Society of Japan, 142*(12), 1371–1377. https://doi.org/10.1248/yakushi.22-00153

Zahiruddin, S., Basist, P., Parveen, A., Parveen, R., Khan, W., Gaurav, G., & Ahmad, S. (2020). Ashwagandha in brain disorders: A review of recent developments. *Journal of Ethnopharmacology, 257*, 112876. https://doi.org/10.1016/j.jep.2020.112876

Made in the USA
Las Vegas, NV
11 November 2024